Every
Body
Should
Know This

Every
Body
Should
Know This

The Science of Eating
for a Lifetime of Health

DR FEDERICA AMATI

MICHAEL  JOSEPH

PENGUIN MICHAEL JOSEPH

UK | USA | Canada | Ireland | Australia
India | New Zealand | South Africa

Penguin Michael Joseph is part of the Penguin Random House group of companies
whose addresses can be found at global.penguinrandomhouse.com

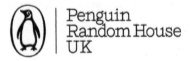

First published 2024
002

Set in 13.5/16pt Garamond MT Std
Typeset by Jouve (UK), Milton Keynes
Printed and bound in Great Britain by Clays Ltd, Elcograf S.p.A.

The authorized representative in the EEA is Penguin Random House Ireland,
Morrison Chambers, 32 Nassau Street, Dublin D02 YH68

A CIP catalogue record for this book is available from the British Library

HARDBACK ISBN: 978–0–241–67961–6
TRADE PAPERBACK ISBN: 978–0–241–66333–2

www.greenpenguin.co.uk

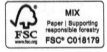

To my beloved daughters;
becoming your mother made me
fall in love with the wonders of the
human body.

Contents

CONTENTS

Preface

Why I Wrote This Book

Growing up, my parents had a nickname for me which was at least partly affectionate. It was *'maestrina'* which translates from the Italian for 'little teacher', and they would call me that because I loved nothing more than sharing my knowledge on my latest discovery or learning – constantly sharing it at every opportunity with anyone who would listen (regardless of whether they were interested or not). As any parent of a young child knows, there are hundreds of discoveries and learnings every day, so I can imagine now, as a parent myself, that the constant updates from me were quite tiring. My beloved nonna on my father's side was a teacher and she adored me as much as I did her, so I relished my label of *maestrina* as it brought me closer to her. I also loved writing stories, mostly starring one of the various pets from our menagerie-style household, and sharing them. Hindsight is a beautiful thing, so looking back now my work as a nutrition educator and scientific writer seems a natural evolution. But the real inspiration to write this book came from the people that I work with.

My job as a nutritionist is to facilitate a better understanding of the importance of one of our daily requirements: the food we all need to eat to survive. Bringing back the connection with our food, the pleasure it can bring and its role as an ally, not an enemy, is often the biggest step in my one-to-one work. Being a nutrition educator, I have the privilege and responsibility of communicating the impact which our diet has on health, longevity and disease to a huge variety of people, from medical students to schools, community centres, journalists, executives and fellow scientists.

I'm sitting in my office, listening to one of my clients tell me about her usual diet; how she feels tired every single day, doesn't recognize herself in the mirror and thinks that her perception of herself and her actual self feel like two separate people. She's disconnected with her body, the food she eats is never a pleasure and it's doing nothing to nourish her physically or mentally. In fact, she feels that her body is constantly letting her down; she exercises to try and reach a specific number on the scale but it remains elusive to her. This is our first session and my main aim is to understand her, her context and her wishes. She is embarking on fertility treatment which is a huge emotional, physical and financial investment. I am part of her team and I take that role very seriously.

Together we explore how and why food can have such an impact on her ovulation, the quality of her eggs, the success of her fertility treatment and the future health of herself and her possible children. On our third consultation a few months into the changes she is implementing, she is feeling much better; she's stopped weighing herself every day, she actually enjoys food for the first time in her adult life and she *feels* better in her own body. Her blood markers have improved and her doctors are happy with her progress and ready to begin treatment. I tell her about the impact of her ovulatory cycle on her metabolism, prepare her for the likely impacts of the drugs she will be taking and reassure her that her nutritional status is now in a much better place for her to begin her journey. She looks at me and says in her melodious Scottish accent: 'You know, Fede, you've changed my life. I just feel like everybody should know this.' And so the seed for this book, already noted on my wish list of things I might do when I grow up, was firmly planted, inspired by the clients I've worked with at all stages of their lives and their resounding positive feedback for how empowering having nutrition as a tool is for them. The research and innovation constantly evolving in the field of nutrition is encouraging, and continues to reinforce the power that food holds over our well-being. My desire is to help more people learn how to create their own unique toolkit for a longer, healthier life through daily food choices as their biggest ally for long-term health and happiness. Crucially, I want to communicate the importance of a life-course approach, because we all live in a complex continuum looking after ourselves and loved ones at different stages.

Another one of my favourite clients is a gentleman in his early sixties. His wife came to see me and essentially convinced him that he too should book an appointment. At first, he was sceptical of what I could possibly teach him about eating for better health. The face of a man who has essentially been sent to see me by a partner is always amusing: polite but definitely straight-faced and not keen on discussing gut health. In this case, a Mediterranean man, he was deeply connected to the food he loved and felt that he was in good nick for his age, essentially not really needing my insight. His results showed that there was room for improvement for his specific goal and we started working together. He followed my advice closely, even quitting a decades-long smoking habit in the process, and now he actually enjoys eating lentils and beans daily; something he visibly smirked at on Day 1. His health markers have improved in ways that frankly neither of us expected, and he and his lovely wife are both feeling better and achieving their health goals together.

Every person I've worked with has taught me something new about humans. It's easy to stay in academia and research aspects of public health, analyse millions of people's data, come to evidence-based conclusions and design interventions that *should* work. In theory we all know what works and doesn't work: we know that we should eat more vegetables, move more, make sure we get enough sleep. A lot of the wisdom inherited from generations of traditions is scientifically sound when it comes to foods and diets. There are common themes from around the globe that carry strong similarities and truths: seasonal local plants are best, eating whole fruits is good for you, fermenting foods helps them keep for longer, going for a *passeggiata* (leisurely stroll) after a meal, sitting with family to eat a homemade meal as a daily non-negotiable. I am Italian so a lot of my examples are from that part of the world, but I will draw similarities and I'm sure readers will find even more in their own lived experience and cultural heritage.

I've always been interested in the human body. As a child in the early 1990s when screentime recommendations weren't a parenting concern, I remember watching a cartoon that depicted all the different functions in the body with little cartoon characters, and I would watch absolutely fascinated that so much could be going on inside of us. I was very young and took to experimenting with some of the learnings by, for example, not brushing my teeth for a week to see if cavities really would form (one did, of course, and I learned not to experiment so freely on myself following the pretty traumatic trip to the dentist). I was lucky to grow up in Italy for the first seven years of my life, so my food environment was naturally full of extra virgin olive oil, seasonal fruits and vegetables and relatively few ultra-processed foods (UPFs). That has unfortunately changed for most children, especially in the UK and the US, where 65 per cent of their daily energy intake comes from UPFs.[1]

UPFs have flooded our supermarkets and our news outlets. Dozens of studies have been published looking at the impact of UPFs on health, across different age groups and looking at different health outcomes. Studies looking at what components of UPFs might be most harmful have also increased, with more research interest on emulsifiers and artificial sweeteners, for example, and an intense debate around whether the definition of UPFs is actually helpful or not. The essence of the argument is that UPFs are industrially made, pre-packaged foods with artificial additives that would be impossible to make at home. I have been quite vocal about the fact that arguing about the definition of UPFs seems futile, when all of the existing evidence clearly points to them being unhealthy. These foods are making up more than half of our daily energy intake. Let's concentrate on reducing their presence on our plates before we engage in debate on whether baked beans should be demonized or not. Baked beans are not the most commonly eaten UPFs so focusing on them is a distraction.

Our grandmothers were right about a lot of things. Every year, science advances in understanding why these things work: fibre in vegetables improves the population of gut bugs that live in our large intestine, and they make important chemicals for us; making sure we get enough sleep gives our bodies and brains an opportunity to clear out unwanted by-products and toxins through the lymphatic and glymphatic system; extra virgin olive oil is the best fat to cook and eat because it has a unique combination of beneficial fatty acids and much higher beneficial plant chemical content than any other fat or oil. I will always remember my maternal grand-mother turning her nose up at the pre-packaged '*schifezze*' (loosely translates to 'yucky things') my brother and I would sometimes be seen eating from a packet. She would gesticu-late and say, 'Eat some real food if you're hungry.' She wasn't wrong, and there are more pre-packaged foods in our diets now than there have ever been.

Teaching medical students at Imperial College London as the nutrition lead for the lifestyle medicine and prevention module (LMAP) keeps me creative in my ability to make epidemiological data compelling. Most undergraduate stu-dents glaze over at the mention of 'epidemiology' and 'data', so storytelling is key. I think the reasons to make nutrition a priority are pretty compelling: 1 in 5 deaths globally could be prevented with improved diets. And 80% of chronic diseases could be prevented by diet and lifestyle changes. That statistic alone is mind-blowing and it warrants re-reading; there is no other single lifestyle change that can so drastically reduce the risk of death and disease for the entire world population. The biggest killers are heart disease, cancer and metabolic diseases. All the biggest killers are driven by three main factors: cigarette smoking, sedentary lifestyles and diet. Our diet encompasses so many things! It is far beyond single nutrients and individual meals; it's a pattern of behaviours and foods that change day to day, month to month and over our life course. From increasing fruit and vegetable consumption (great) and adding beans and pulses to our plates (excellent), to drinking too much alcohol (not good) and having too much added salt and sugar in pre-prepared foods (bad), it also contributes to time spent with friends and family as a crucial social activity and informs how we interact with our environment and other living creatures. It is complex and never static; our diet evolves with us as individuals, within family units and in wider communities.

When we moved to London, I have clear memories of boxes of cereal bars and bottles of bright orange squash served at break time at my new school. Not only was I confused by them as they didn't look like food; they also weren't as obviously delicious as the pre-packed cake snacks popular in Italy, so I found them completely unappealing fake food alternatives. I was very lucky to have a brilliant education and parents – Mum a medical doctor and regulatory scientist, Dad an electronic engineer and inventor – who let me follow my own path despite it being a bit different. I always loved science: biology especially, chemistry not so much, but our relationship improved when I went on to study pharmacology. I also loved English literature and history and I refused to drop them, leaving school with a smorgasbord of A-levels and a love for writing, as well as science and learning.

Nutrition science has reached an exciting tipping point. There has never been so much interest in the power of food for health and we have unprecedented access to technology and data to help us understand the details of what makes us unique. With a simple-to-use app, we can log the foods we eat, understand their composition and track how our dietary choices make us feel, how they impact our health and how we can improve. Personalized nutrition and understanding the nuances of the gut microbiome are within reach, and the next frontier is to weave all these strands together into a story across the whole life spectrum. This book addresses the phases of this spectrum, the life course, and what we know about each stage. We will discover the exciting power which food has to help us thrive throughout those changes.

In my time studying and researching at universities from my teens to today, I have learned so much – and contributed to some – science. It's been a passion of mine from the start to communicate what I learn, to transmit some of the wonder I have felt in discovering how our bodies work, how we can help them and what changes our health over time. This book is dedicated to making the story of our bodies' relationship with food more accessible, so everybody can have a better insight into what works for them personally, and reclaim the pleasure and the power of food.

Introduction

What's the Problem, Doc?

The food we eat impacts our body day after day and week after week, building into dietary patterns we often carry with us for months and years and pass down generations. Looking at our overall dietary pattern of what foods we eat as a powerful indicator of health is an empowering concept. It is much easier to know which foods to eat more of, rather than focus our energy on individual meal composition and learning how to count abstract things like macros and calories. Aside from table sugar, there is no food I can think of which is fairly represented by its caloric and macronutrient content, and even with sugar, how it impacts our bodies varies hugely from person to person and it varies from time to time in the same person. This is where I hope to bring a new lens on nutrition and health. Our life course is a marathon, not a sprint, and what we need to thrive changes depending on which mile we are running.

Understanding our story as individuals is so important, but there are a few things which virtually every person has to do to survive every day. Many more things are needed to thrive, but survival really relies on five main pillars: breathing, sleeping, nourishment, movement and socializing. In that order, a person can survive a few minutes without breathing, a few days without water, a fortnight or so without eating or sleeping and a variable length of time without movement or human contact. We know from the current loneliness epidemic in elderly adults living alone in the UK, that having no social contact can hugely impact health, quality of life and even longevity. Prisoners in solitary confinement have an increased risk of premature death, and some very cruel studies in the 1800s confirmed the importance of socializing, when they observed that children die if you starve them of social contact, even when everything else is provided.

So far, so obvious, of course, but isn't it curious how our education system and our lifestyle so often overlook these five fundamental needs? In the past five years, there has been a renewed interest in human biology and how we can improve our lives, no doubt partly inspired by the shock that we lived through during the COVID-19 pandemic. From books about instant weight loss and strict rules on how to live your life for ultimate financial success, there was a new surge in books about connecting to our mental health, using our breath to reduce anxiety, how to grow our own food and how to look after our sleep.

And about time too; our children receive no formal education on how to look after their basic needs, and as adults we are lucky if we have any more insight. Even medical students only started receiving formal education on nutrition, mental health and the impact of social inequalities, sleep and physical activity in the past decade – I know, because I teach them at one of the best universities in the world, and they only have a few hours with me to cover nutrition. If the vast majority of our current doctors, nurses, health visitors, mid-wives, teachers and politicians don't have access to fundamental training for a basic understanding of nutrition science, it is perhaps not that surprising that our food environment and diet-related health outcomes are all steadily worsening (spoiler alert: most of the chronic diseases that afflict us as we age are related to poor nutrition).

Epidemiology is the study of whole populations and the trends we observe in both risk factors and disease outcomes. For example, epidemiological studies have analysed the relationship between coffee consumption and cancer (protective) and the risk of alcohol consumption and breast cancer (increases, especially in post-menopausal women). The key caveat to epidemiological studies is that they can only observe associations on which we can then base *theories* for causation. Because epidemiological studies observe people over time with different lifestyles, different levels of consumption of the 'exposure' – coffee and alcohol as examples – and don't always have detailed biochemical markers to accompany the analysis, using instead outcomes such as 'death' or 'cancer diagnosis', we can be confident of biologically plausible associations, but we can't infer causation from them.

Biological plausibility is what is sometimes missing from interpretations of associations. For something to be biologically plausible, there has to be a clear mechanism for it to take place. For example, it is biologically plausible that drinking too much wine in the evening will cause me to feel tired the next day, as alcohol is a well-understood toxin which impacts many processes in our bodies, making us feel a bit crap. It is harder to find a biological plausibility for things that have no clear mechanism to connect them. In epidemiology lectures it's always fun to show graphs of how the number of films starring Nicolas Cage correlates with the number of people who drowned in pools. Obviously, Nicolas Cage movies don't have any relationship to swimming pool drowning incidents (or do they?!), but seriously, the same level of common biological and physiological sense is not often applied to health, and especially nutrition. If there is no plausible mechanism whereby an exposure (Nicolas Cage movies) and the outcome (swimming pool drownings) are associated, we should not assume causation. There are millions of other factors that are likely to play more important roles.

FIGURE 1. The correlation between number of people who drowned by falling into a pool and films Nicolas Cage appeared in.

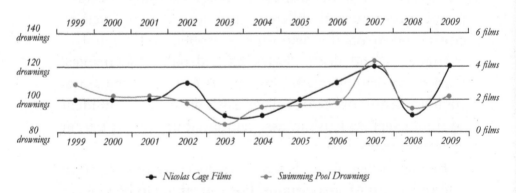

But I digress. What I really want to focus on is the power which dietary change has to alleviate our current global health crisis. We are moving towards a population where 1 in 2 adults are overweight or obese, 1 in 3 children are the same,

1 in 2 of us will at some point develop cancer in our lives and 1 in 5 will experience poor mental health. This means that in each household there is likely to be multimorbidity (the presence of two or more long-term health conditions such as heart disease and type 2 diabetes) at any one time, and in a rapidly ageing population, prioritizing a longer *health span* is critical. Globally, 1 in 5 deaths could be prevented with better nutrition. And what is more interesting to us as individuals is the power which our daily food choices hold in preventing disability and ill health. It's hard to have a conversation with an adult of any age who doesn't report some sort of ailment, from the more obvious diet-associated conditions like type 2 diabetes and obesity, to depression, anxiety, inflammatory diseases, allergies, heart disease, stroke, constipation, bloating and thyroid dysfunctions. All of these conditions affect quality of life in varying degrees and can lead to increasingly serious disability and illness as they progress. Nutrition plays a dual role in both being able to reduce the risk of developing these, and in managing symptoms effectively to reduce their impact on our lives and the lives of our loved ones.

One thing we all have in common is food. We need it to survive, it surrounds us everywhere and the food we choose to eat has direct consequences on our health and our happiness. But we have lost touch with our food; it's produced far away from our day-to-day lives and arrives prepared and prepacked to our homes, our desks and our stores. We have built a food environment that is based on food marketing and arbitrary targets instead of responding to our biological needs and nourishing ourselves as individuals. We aren't well equipped to navigate this for ourselves, and those who are in positions of food power often aren't either. To top it off, the food industry is hardly regulated in the claims it can make or the way it can advertise its products, so we are bombarded with marketing designed to encourage us to consume more of what is eventually making us ill.

A report published in 2023 by Tortoise Media on the current state of our food environment revealed that 70 per cent of the food produced for our supermarket shelves is UPF. A handful of food manufacturing companies in the UK make *exclusively* UPFs. The price per calorie of UPFs is significantly cheaper than minimally processed or unprocessed foods made by the same company. All of these points paint a damning picture of profit over people, but as the food industry is a free market for profit-making, who should be reining this in? We'll be hard pressed to find many shareholders applying pressure to reduce profits, at least momentarily, in order to improve public health. And so we live in a food environment that is bursting with easy-to-eat, delicious, conveniently packaged, brightly coloured UPFs that are meticulously tested to be as moreish as possible and not filling. The more we eat, the better the bottom line, and the science that goes into making these foods so successful is excellent.

It doesn't have to be this way, of course. A documentary which I helped to pull together for BBC *Panorama* working with Tim Spector and Sarah Berry as leading voices, highlighted the dangers of UPFs on our health both in the long term and in the short term, thanks to the lovely Twins-UK volunteers who let us run a mini-trial with them. It is often shocking to people to realize how much of our children's food is UPFs and the damage it is likely doing to their developing bodies and minds. But other countries are doing better than us in the UK and the US. Italy and Romania, for example, have much lower consumption of UPFs: around 15 per cent of daily calorie consumption instead of 50–65 per cent in the UK population. On average, the majority of the food we eat in the UK comes from UPFs, and the higher percentages come from data we have on children's diets. We have to learn from the countries that are still doing better than us (for now), and prioritize making fresh, dried and frozen, whole or minimally processed foods a priority. We can introduce restrictions on marketing to children, just like we did by removing cartoon characters from breakfast cereals. We can also help restore our understanding of food and how essential it is for us and our health by reclaiming a sense of pride and priority for mealtimes, whether at home, school or work.

In my clinical practice, my clients often tell me that they can't believe they don't know more about the importance of food before coming to me for advice. By the time they get to me, they have tried a few things, including severe calorie restriction, and they have the means to pay for my time, so they are the tip of the iceberg. They tell me they have no idea what they're supposed to eat any more and that the scientific debate around food is so confusing that they don't know where to turn. My job as a medical scientist and a nutritionist is to cut through the noise with solid evidence-based advice and help people reconnect with their food and, most importantly, themselves.

When I am invited to give talks for communities, I am always touched by the stories. Recently, a woman at a wonderful community centre in London where I gave a talk on the gut microbiome, told me of her despair as she was trying to help her husband with a severe, debilitating psoriasis that had taken over his whole body. The doctors at A&E where he went for help, as he was so desperate with his burning skin in the summer heat, gave him cortisone cream and told him it is a chronic condition he needed to learn to live with. His skin worsened and cracked and burned with the cortisone and he had to take time off work, which his family couldn't afford. I learned that he had fatty liver disease, a condition known to increase the risk of psoriasis, and yet he had received no advice on how to change his diet to help resolve this. He was drinking several sugary energy drinks every day and had not been told to try and stop doing that, or that simply eating more fruits and vegetables could help him. This is not to say that the A&E doctors did anything wrong, of course – I am only too aware of the mounting pressures on the NHS and junior doctors – but there are millions of people who could see an immediate improvement to their health with nutrition education that isn't widely available.

What's disheartening is that only a tiny proportion of people can access specialists like me, and those people are often the more fortunate, more affluent ones who have the resources and the referrals to access nutrition advice. It's no secret that nutrition drives a huge wedge in the health disparity we see in the UK and the US; the richest households have the lowest risk of nutrition-related diseases like obesity, whereas the poorest households have growing risk year on year, and this difference in risk is most noticeable for children. That's why the headline news of 'Number of UK children with obesity has reached a plateau' actually hides the true distribution of 'UK children in richest households are at reduced risk of obesity whilst poorest children's risk continues to grow.'

Do I think nutrition education is the magic bullet to ending food inequality and health disparity? No (though maybe I did at twenty-two!), but I do think that there is a level of understanding, which I have included in this book, that we could all universally benefit from. And if one doctor, teacher, nurse, politician, parent, nursery school teacher, grandmother, shopkeeper, restaurant owner or social media influencer decides to pass this information on, then the ripple effect of this book will be worth it. If it helps people prioritize and support politicians and those in power who care about our food environment then it can be part of the health revolution for the future of our children and our planet. This desire to spread the word on the importance of good nutrition is also what drives my passion working with ZOE, the nutrition science company. ZOE's actual company mission is to *improve the health of millions* and we truly do aspire to do this by providing excellent nutrition education through published research, the app, the podcasts, social media and the wonderful content that is thoroughly and carefully researched and written and cross-checked. We have reached over one million people already and that makes me so proud.

Welcome to your body

We all care about how we feel today and many of us want to give our future selves a helping hand. The food we eat has an immediate impact on us (even before we take a bite!) and the pattern of food we eat over our lifetime is one of the strongest predictors for our future health. As far as preparing for the future is concerned, investing in our food choices is the simplest and most secure guaranteed return of investment available to us. It's bound to have a positive impact. In this first-of-a-kind book, nutrition, medical science and public health come together to create a simple, evidence-based guide to what we should all know and love about food and how it affects us.

It all starts with understanding more about ourselves and learning to reconnect with our innate wisdom. Human bodies are wondrous, exciting holobionts* that have evolved to survive with the trillions of microorganisms who call us home. Each of us is as complex as the entire universe, with each specific function in each one of our cells perfectly honed to work towards the common goal of survival of the species. With all of this wonder, complexity and endless discovery (we still don't know much about most of the trillions of microbes that we evolved with or the 98 per cent of our genome that is 'non-coding') comes one powerful realization: what we need to thrive is already inside us. All we need to do is understand the basics and understand our individual selves; the rest has been done for us by evolution.

Working with children, as well as having my own, has been one of my greatest joys and educational experiences. Babies express their needs until they are met, infants relish the

---

* From the *Collins English Dictionary*: a holobiont is any agglomeration of a host and related organisms that functions as a discrete ecological unit.

experience of trying new foods presented as safe by their parents, toddlers will not eat if they are not hungry and they will let you know when they are. Hunger, thirst, tiredness, desire for movement, need for connection: young children and infants have not learned to suppress these drives and they don't have the neurocognitive ability to do so. They learn how to cope with stress from us, learn how to delay gratification from us, and they also learn when to override their nutrition cues from us. Insisting that children eat when they aren't hungry, or learn not to eat when they are, is the first step in losing that connection with our individual nutritional needs. My primary school didn't allow us to leave the dining table until we had finished all the food on our plates. I often hear well-meaning parents tell their children, 'You can't be hungry! No, no more food, you've had enough,' signalling to the child that their interpretation of their hunger is incorrect. This is the result of societal conditioning and not any one individual's fault, of course. Diet culture plays its huge part in all of this, and I like to think that our children will be in a better place than I was growing up in the 1990s when drinking water to quell your hunger and the coffee, apple and cigarette diet were widely accepted solutions.

The majority of my adult clients have become so preoccupied with what to eat, they have lost the love for food. Many of them have had decades of a troubled or problematic relationship with food, trying to cut out entire food groups or suppressing their appetite as much as they could – usually in the pursuit of being thin. This has left them confused about what to eat, at worst completely disassociated with the importance of food and overwhelmed at the constant noise and contradictory advice available in all corners of the internet, podcasts and traditional media. I am not saying I have all the answers, nobody does. But I do think that having a fundamental understanding of a few basic principles can really help to evaluate whether the latest surprising update is likely to be impactful or not. The first part of the book is all about the key principles, before we dive into the changes that make us all unique in applying these principles to our own decision-making.

This book is a manual about eating for life; it doesn't 'dive deep' into any one area or condition. It is designed to tell a story of food as our ally for health through a life-course approach, touching on the biggest 'windows of opportunity' that human development offers us: the key moments in time when our physiology, our metabolism and our needs for certain foods change, which also makes them uniquely powerful moments for us to change our relationship with food.

Each stage of life is relevant to every body. You will have lived through the initial stages – the first 1,000 days and beyond – by the time you're reading this book. Regardless of age, everyone has known and loved somebody at each stage of the life course first-hand, yet many of us have had no food education whatsoever to navigate the changes, despite the crucial role of nutrition. First, we have conception, pregnancy and the first two years of life. Also known as the first 1,000 days, this is a woefully under-appreciated golden window of opportunity where diet impacts the life of the mother and her baby (or babies). Infancy and childhood hold an incredibly important place in forming the blueprint for future health, and the science investigating this stage of life is incredibly powerful and has produced extremely compelling evidence that we should be investing in this time.

In later childhood and adolescence, we have windows in growth spurts, hormonal changes and important brain structure changes which require extra special attention. Adolescents are largely underserved by science and by society, despite their pivotal role in shaping the immediate future. In Parts 2 and 3 we look at how improving nutrition in our reproductive years can help to prevent the insidious onset of mental health problems, autoimmune and metabolic diseases, which are all consistently increasing.

The final three parts of this book are dedicated to the ultimate 'life goals' population: the healthy elders who have *lived* past midlife, not simply aged beyond it. Most of us will (hopefully) spend the majority of our lives in this part of the book, older than 50 and younger than 120 – that is quite the age-bracket! And yet most of us don't understand the changing needs that living longer brings. That includes scientists, because living this long is a recent phenomenon which we are rapidly investigating and trying to understand.

What this book won't offer is any promise of biohacking, any route to guaranteed immortality or any advice to help with looking twenty in your eighties. I firmly believe that living a long and healthy life is a privilege to be cherished and not feared, masked or avoided. I also believe that to imagine ourselves as capable of outsmarting the process of ageing is extremely arrogant and ignorant – we haven't yet understood so much of the complexity that makes us human; to think we've mastered a machine/supplement/treatment/protocol that can stop nature doing its thing is simply ludicrous.

The key fundamentals

There are some almost universal truths which we currently understand about our bodies and our metabolism. This forms the basis of how we understand food in a fundamental way: building blocks, energy, pleasure, repair, movement, and removal of by-products or toxins. All of the foods we find in nature, which grow from the ground or have eaten things that grow from the ground, have a combination of these elements. Some foods supply us with more building blocks (proteins and fats), others with more energy (carbohydrates and fats), and others still with more elements to repair and remove toxins (fibre and plant chemicals). Small amounts of electrolytes and minerals such as sodium and copper are found in various foods and are needed for the healthy function of our nervous system and connective tissue structure as two examples. What's fundamental to understand at this point is that most whole foods contain a majority if not all of these elements in different proportions, and our body absorbs, breaks down, repackages and distributes them to where they are needed and can also create its own version of some of them.

Understanding just how well equipped our body is for surviving with much less food than we have access to today is really important. We have evolved, over millions of years, to survive and reproduce on an unpredictable combination and abundance of foods. This is why our liver, a magical organ, can literally create things for us: it can create glucose, it can create proteins, it can create fats! It takes pieces from what we feed it (or from our stored goodies) and then builds

FIGURE 2. Overlapping macronutrient contents in our foods.

MACRONUTRIENTS

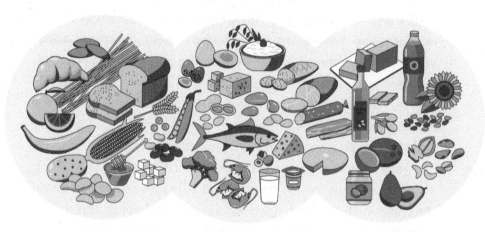

CARBOHYDRATES   PROTEINS   FATS

what we need. Like a Lego magician, our liver deconstructs and rebuilds what is needed from what we have available to us. Alongside the liver, our gut microbes also create useful Lego from the foods we eat. Eating a variety of nutrient-dense foods ensures our Lego stores are well stocked for every day and tomorrow's building work.

With this in mind, it's easier to understand how eating a variety of different foods could be helpful: the more types of Lego pieces we provide, the more interesting and colourful a construction we can make. If we survive on the same food every day, as happens in people with severe food phobias who can eat just one or a small handful of specific food for years, our liver runs out of ways to make all the different components needed to thrive, and gut microbes only make a limited amount of helpful pieces. Before we know it, we are suffering with deficiencies which lead to a loss of function and health.

This is also linked to the fact that there are some things we can't make for ourselves: plant chemicals also known as micro-nutrients or phytochemicals. Some essential amino acids, vitamins and minerals, from tryptophan and vitamin A to iron, potassium and magnesium, are needed in very small quantities, but they have to come from our food and are essential for health. We can actually make our own vitamin D, vitamin K and vitamin B12, thanks to our skin cells and gut microbes, but as a general rule, we need to eat a variety of nutrients. The thing is that eating a variety of foods, especially those that grow from the soil, which contains many of the essential micro and macro nutrients, can easily provide the majority of what we need.

Another universal truth is that our cells work by using glu-cose as fuel to power the tiny batteries called mitochondria that live inside our cells, excluding red blood cells. Mitochon-dria create the power needed for everything from creating new skin cells to orchestrating the way our neurons fire elec-tric impulses and chemical messages across our nervous system, as well as our speedy immune response to a badly grazed knee. It's easy to get sucked in to mitochondrial sci-ence, and there are some brilliant books on the topic, but for the purpose of day-to-day life and health I like to keep some perspective and focus on how the overall machine is work-ing, not just the batteries. It's important to understand the crucial role glucose plays in every single cellular function to appreciate why our body is so programmed to seek and eat foods that contain it: it plays a massive role in our metabol-ism and metabolic health precisely because it's essential.

So we absorb food and break it down into its useful pieces, we are able to build our own useful pieces given a few essential components are provided, and our cells are powered by glucose. Another universal truth is that we don't absorb food straight into our bloodstream. I'll go as far as to say that we aren't designed to receive nutrients directly into our bloodstream, and IV drips used outside of a medical setting can be problematic. Our digestive system and liver work very hard to selectively break down, transport, package and redistribute every single morsel and gulp of everything that passes our lips. Starting from our mouth where digestion begins, our microbes not only work to break down and create nutrients and chemicals for us; they work hard to analyse any possible disease-causing bug or toxin and communicate with our immune system, waving microbial red flags if they find something untoward. This process doesn't always work perfectly, and its complexity also makes it prone to glitches such as food allergies.

The final fundamental which underpins so much of our biology is the concept of homeostasis. The word comes from the two Greek words *homoios* and *stasis*, which roughly translate to 'stay the same'. The term 'homeostasis' was first coined by the physiologist Walter Bradford Cannon in the early twentieth century. Cannon used this term to describe the body's ability to maintain a stable internal environment despite changes in external conditions. Homeostasis involves various physiological processes that help to regulate and balance the internal environment of the body, including temperature, pH, fluid balance, and concentrations of various electrolytes and nutrients. I can't stress enough how fundamental this concept is, and if you stop reading this book after this page then that's OK, because homeostasis busts so many nutrition and health myths, and it's key to understanding biological plausibility.

Let's start with one of my favourite examples: the pH levels in our body. A common myth that refuses to die is the idea that we can somehow change our body's pH level by drinking 'alkaline' water or taking 'alkaline supplements'. Now, if we consider the fact that our body's pH differs from organ to organ, with an incredibly low (acidic) pH in our stomach which is literally filled with hydrochloric acid, to the very alkaline bile salts directly after the stomach produced by the gall bladder, the idea that we need to alkalize everything is obviously counterintuitive. But let's go back to homeostasis – our body works very hard to maintain the correct pH level in every tissue and at cellular level. This is because, as we've just seen, different cells in the body need to be at different pH levels to function properly. If our pH levels really were to all magically change to the level we're supposed to be at (alkaline according to some), we would probably die. Hence the idea that trying to change our pH level through a well-marketed 'alkaline' water (pH typically around 7 or very much neutral for those interested), gulping down lemon water first thing in the morning (acidic at around pH 3.5), or indeed a specific supplement of any sort, is a slap in the face to the intelligence of our intricately designed physiology.

Hopefully I've convinced you that an understanding of how our body works is not only interesting but also useful, and that the way forward is filled with joy, empathy for ourselves and an appreciation of the journey of life itself. In the next sections we will explore food and its impact across different parts of life, and I'll bring in some examples and stories from my own experience as well as those I am lucky to work with. Major scientific studies, published works and recommended resources are referenced at the end for those who want to learn more. Simple tips and advice which I find help the majority of my clients are also included in this book, with the hope that more people can start to make positive changes to their nutrition, and put much needed pressure on those shaping our food environment to do the same.

Understanding nutrition science

The world of nutrition is probably the noisiest of all the sciences. You don't get as many people weighing in with their opinions on breathing and sleep, the other common human practices, and very few people claim to be experts in the field. Exercise and movement used to have a similar problem, where family members, Hollywood stars and Olympians all had similar platforms to express their own ideas on the topic. But nowadays, I definitely feel nutrition misinformation, overwhelming opinions and quackery is at its peak. Or at least I hope we're near the peak, because it's the wildest notions that make it to the fore of public debate.

One of the best tools we have to help navigate the confusion is to have a scientific approach. Always ask questions, don't automatically assume that because someone said something it must be true. Even if they are very senior or sound very convincing, an open mind will always welcome questions, and challenging ideas is essential to scientific debate. So the first thing to look out for is somebody who is not willing to be challenged or to engage in debate. That isn't a good sign.

The second thing about science is that it evolves and changes. And nutrition science specifically is evolving incredibly rapidly. A good example of this is the long-held belief that eating cholesterol-rich foods would increase blood cholesterol levels. We now know this not to be the case – fatty acids are much more important[1] – but for decades government bodies recommended that people not eat eggs, shellfish and sardines despite them being nutrient-rich foods. I think we are getting to a stage where some key factors are beyond doubt, and these changes are normally in the detail. For example, we know that eating food in its whole form, with as little industrial processing as possible, is good for us.

There's a lot of noise trying to sell us other foods with marketing budgets that make Mariah Carey appear affordable, with branding that distracts us and entices us to buy the latest high-protein, keto friendly, gluten free, agave nectar bar so we forget that the humble chickpea or cabbage are actually brilliant foods to eat. There is no scientific controversy about the health benefits of whole foods, and I would bet my bottom dollar that there won't be a 180-degree change on that point. There is still ongoing debate about smaller details like are emulsifiers worse than artificial sweeteners? Are all artificial sweeteners bad? Should we worry about baked beans as a UPF? To me, all of these factors are white noise when considering the bigger picture, and the scientific stance on them is likely to change in the coming years. It won't change the premise that eating whole foods prepared at home is better for us.

Many of us don't choose to study science past the age of fourteen. It isn't for everyone, but there are some key tools that we use as scientists to understand how much weight to give to evidence, which can be really useful. The evidence pyramid, a version of which is below, outlines the hierarchy of evidence. In most cases, ideas start at the bottom of the pyramid and work their way up. If the idea is a solid one and it does in fact work out to be evidence based, it can take quite a few years to get there as each step requires time to prove the idea.

For example, an expert might think that gut microbes are having an effect on human health. This expert opinion is

FIGURE 3. The hierarchy of evidence pyramid.

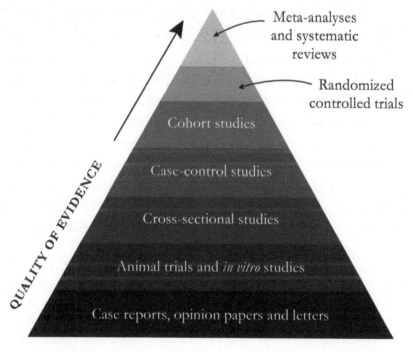

Meta-analyses and systematic reviews

Randomized controlled trials

Cohort studies

Case-control studies

Cross-sectional studies

Animal trials and *in vitro* studies

Case reports, opinion papers and letters

QUALITY OF EVIDENCE

unlikely to shift anyone's attitude to gut health or the micro-biome, and so the expert embarks on a series of studies to try and unpick his idea further. The first step might be to look at animal studies; these studies and the ones conducted 'in vitro' (i.e. in a test tube) are used to see whether it's plausible that a mechanism for the idea exists.* He starts testing micro-biome differences in hundreds of identical twins and showing that, despite being genetic clones, they have unique microbial signatures (these twins are in what we call a cohort study).

Next, the scientist, together with other scientists inter-ested in this topic, designs a cohort study to test how much impact the gut microbiome has on health outcomes by fol-lowing people up over time (prospective study); this is important because you have to wait and see what happens, even if that ends up going against your initial theory. In this example, the scientist is Professor Tim Spector and the cohort study is the PREDICT 1 study. The study showed significant differences in individual responses to the same test meal, and the gut microbiome was found to differ in a way that is likely to make it a mediator for those differences. This study was the first of many that went on to form the basis for ZOE, the personalized nutrition company.

The next step up on the ladder is Randomized controlled trials (RCT), which are expensive to run and need meticulous planning. A good RCT can have a huge impact on the

---

* In-vitro studies are often used as 'evidence' for supplements and their health benefits. We are not test tubes; just because a specific chemical halts cancer cells in a glass container, it does not mean this will take place in our complex, multi-system, intelligent bodies.

understanding of a topic. ZOE ran an RCT to test its own product for efficacy. In a study called the METHOD trial, people were randomized to either receive the full ZOE experience or standard dietary advice with added support. This is a way to really test whether ZOE (or another intervention like a drug or specific diet) can improve measurable health outcomes in an impactful way. Again, Tim and the rest of the science team didn't know what would happen, but with good quality RCTs they have to be registered and there is a duty to publish results whether they are positive or negative. METHOD found that people following ZOE advice did have clinically impactful improvements to their health, including massive improvements to their gut microbiome.

As more RCTs are done to answer the same question – does personalized nutrition work, and is the gut microbiome important for health? – we start to see a clearer answer. Eventually, when there is enough data, a review can be conducted which gathers all the data from all the different trials, weighs it up and assigns a score of how likely the intervention (in this case personalized nutrition) is to have a positive or negative effect on health outcomes. This process is called a meta-analysis and it sits at the top of the pyramid.

Data is essential to run a meta-analysis; without it, you can't pool and analyse the results. The more data from high-quality studies the better, and the more certain we can be of the evidence. An example of where this is the case is the benefits of a Mediterranean diet as a positive nutrition intervention. The Mediterranean diet, unlike personalized nutrition which is still in its relative infancy, has been studied, analysed and used as an intervention for decades by dozens of research groups on millions of patients. There is so much data on the Mediterranean diet that we now have what's known as a systematic meta-review[2] which is off the top of the pyramid and is an analysis of the analyses!

Anyone who says there isn't enough evidence that any one dietary pattern is likely to reduce the risk of all chronic diseases, including mental health, needs to read through that paper and the many systematic reviews on the Mediterranean diet. The evidence is very strong and there is no real mystery left to it; a diet high in primarily whole foods, vegetables, legumes, whole grains, fruits, nuts and seeds with regular oily fish and extra virgin olive oil consumption, some dairy and eggs and only occasional meat is the framework for a healthy diet. It's called the Me-Di for short and it is comprehensively evidence based.

What's missing on our pyramid is the plethora of other sources of information we have today. YouTube videos, podcasts, documentaries, social media posts, books, blogs, magazines, newspapers and all other consumable media; they don't make it to the pyramid because they aren't evidence. They are opinion and may be discussing evidence, but they don't contribute to our overall understanding of what interventions impact change and how. Some of these may be more evidence based than others and might cite evidence from the scientific literature that does sit in our pyramid. The reason why healthcare professionals are recommended in shared decision-making for your health, is because most healthcare registration requires you to prove that you keep yourself up to date with the evidence base. For example, registered dieticians (RD), AfN accredited nutritionists (ANutr or RNutr), psychotherapists (UKCP registered) and of course medical doctors (MD) have to apply to re-register their professional title every year and prove they have continued their education.

So a registered health professional who is required to undertake continued registration has a duty of care and of keeping up to date. Others don't. Hopefully, by understanding the pyramid of evidence you too can ask questions about where this advice or evidence comes from. Beware the influencer or 'bio-hacker' who claims they don't need to cite evidence for their claims because scientific evidence is rigged. They are probably the most worrying new trend I've come across, and although scientific research is not perfect* it is certainly more robust than hearsay or personal anecdote, and I would say that the overwhelming majority of scientists and researchers have a common goal to improve our understanding and application of science to improve health.

One thing to look out for is when studies are funded by industry bodies. This is particularly relevant when the industry in question is trying to sell a product that is closely implicated with harm. For example, when Coca-Cola pays for studies on health or when British American Tobacco funds research on the benefits of vaping. I'm not saying all research funded by industry is skewed; after all, funding research is really hard and private companies often have the funds to spend so it would be naïve to say this should *never* happen, but it's worth noting that when a collagen supplement funds research on skin improvements, the very positive results

---

* *The Diet Myth* by Tim Spector and *Bad Science* by Ben Goldacre are excellent books on this.

should be taken with a large pinch of salt. It's not necessarily invalid but it isn't impartial.

With everything I've described in this section of the book, whenever you are weighing up a lifestyle or dietary change you are thinking about implementing in your life, consider the following dietary principles; they will help to shape the way you think about food for your health and the planet's health too.

Every Body Should Know This

- One single food or nutrient is not going to be the answer to all ailments. There is no such thing as one 'superfood'.
- UPFs are pervasive on our supermarket shelves and in our homes and they're having a negative impact on our health. Knowing how to identify and reduce them is important.
- Eating foods in their whole form as much as possible and cooking from scratch is a great way to improve our health and learn more about how our food is made.
- Look out for unrealistic claims, superfoods and 'miracle' food solutions. A healthy diet is about a pattern of foods eaten over days, weeks and months. Take a wide-lensed view of the sorts of foods you're eating most of the time, aligning with the Mediterranean/Planetary diet pyramids as much as possible.

FIGURE 4. Mediterranean diet and planetary health double pyramid.

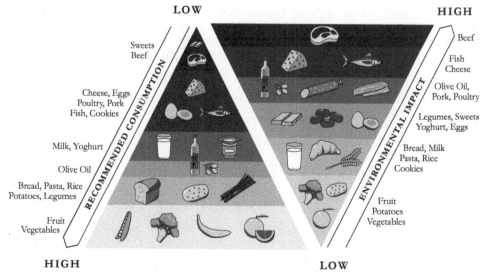

ENVIRONMENTAL PYRAMID

LOW   HIGH

Sweets
Beef

Cheese, Eggs
Poultry, Pork
Fish, Cookies

Milk, Yoghurt

Olive Oil

Bread, Pasta, Rice
Potatoes, Legumes

Fruit
Vegetables

RECOMMENDED CONSUMPTION

ENVIRONMENTAL IMPACT

Beef

Fish
Cheese

Olive Oil,
Pork, Poultry

Legumes, Sweets
Yoghurt, Eggs

Bread, Milk
Pasta, Rice
Cookies

Fruit
Potatoes
Vegetables

HIGH   LOW

FOOD PYRAMID

- The food environment, especially in the US and UK, is designed to maximize profit not health. Being aware of this is the first step in improving our nutrition choices.
- Biological plausibility is really important. If there's no clear mechanism by which something can influence an outcome, they're probably not related. If something seems outrageous, it probably isn't accurate. This ties in with the next point:
- Homeostasis is all powerful. The constant calibration of all our systems to keep our health steady and return things to baseline is how we stay

35

alive. We cannot outsmart our biology; we either work with it and improve our health, spend lots of time and money trying to outsmart it and forget to live, or we ignore it and suffer the consequences.

- Scientific evidence is important. Understanding the basics of how to interpret it can help you untangle fact from fiction and data from anecdote. Having the tools to understand science can give us the agency to make informed decisions by ourselves, without relying on external influences.

PART I

The Golden Window of Opportunity: The First 1,000 Days and Early Years

The first 1,000 days refers to an exact window of time from the day of conception to a child's second birthday. It adds up to 1,000 days (give or take depending on whether a baby is born prematurely or not). The first 1,000 days sounds important and like something we should care about; it has a momentous note to it like an Arnie Schwarzenegger movie about the beginning of time. If only it would get the attention that an Arnie film gets. It is indeed a momentous time when lots of important things happen that would be worthy of posters and expensive adverts on the London tube, yet it's widely unknown and unspoken of outside of the scientific research on the topic (there's lots of that!). I'd love for us all to think about this time of life differently and give it the attention it deserves.

One of my presentations on the first 1,000 days begins with the statement: 'Forty-eight of the fifty-two cell differentiations required to make an adult human are complete by the day of birth.' We all start off as one cell (the egg) that gets kicked into action by another cell (the sperm) and what follows is a series of cell differentiations. This means that the cells change to form the basis of our organs: from brain to eyes to feet, the initial cell has differentiated to make different cells which then divide and make lots of cells that make up our whole body. Forty-eight of the total fifty-two cell differentiations to make a whole adult human with all of the heart, hair, brain, fingers and eyeballs have happened by birth. I find this amazing as it tells us just how much of the scaffolding and building blocks for the rest of our lives is actually created in the womb.

Just a heads up that this is one of the topics I get more passionate about, and it is also one of the most difficult. Whenever I want to shout from the rooftops about the importance of *the first 1,000 days*, the *golden window of opportunity* and the wonderful theories that help us explain just how this period of life is so powerful, I am met with sharp inhales and various degrees of raised eyebrows. Some podcasters have told me, 'We just can't include that information, it's too scary to the public'; publishers have told me, 'Books sold for fertility and pre-conception just don't do very well, unfortunately, there isn't a market for it.' But more fellow scientists, clinicians, parents and certainly my own clients trying to conceive have told me just how important this information is to them. So I'm going with my gut and with what I think is most useful. Sure, it might be scary to realize all of this information at first, I've been there with my own pregnancies. But not knowing doesn't make it go away, and not sharing the information takes away our potential to significantly improve future generations' health. And why on earth would anyone not want to improve things for our children?

Understanding how we are created and what role nutrition plays in building that blueprint for life is fundamental. It helps us understand our risks as adults as well as improving our children's and grandchildren's health. It will almost certainly also make you feel quite strongly about marketing foods to children and new parents. I hope so.

The egg, the sperm and the symphony of life

It starts with an egg. An egg that was already present in your mother's ovaries when she was in her mother's, your grandmother's, womb. This egg carries genetic and epigenetic information passed down from your mother and influenced by your grandmother's choices. The way I like to think of genetics and epigenetics is with an analogy about music: the genes you carry are the musical notes on a music sheet; they are the symphony of life itself waiting to be played. Epigenetics are the annotations added to the notes to describe how they are played and their tempo: *pianissimo* for those soft, gentle parts, *crescendo*, for the dramatic parts. Epigenetic markers are identified by methylation of certain genes which essentially just means an added 'note' on the genes to impact how and when it is played. What about the orchestra and pianist who will be playing this music? Enter the host microbiome – the millions of microbes and their genetic information and products that you begin to accumulate from the moment you are born. Viruses, bacteria, parasites and other tiny creatures who call your body home and play a huge part in your symphony. The concert hall is your body, whose structure too is crucially important, and is affected by maternal diet in a fundamental way.

We can't easily change our genetics, and epigenetic markers are often unpredictable and transient. What we can impact is the structure of the concert hall, how we maintain it, and who the musicians are. And you guessed it, diet is the major player.

Going back to the egg and sperm, the blueprint and the foundations for the concert hall; they take ninety days to mature to their point of meeting. And what a very intense ninety days from germ cell to fully fledged life-making potential! Every conception is a miracle: the chances of a successful meeting between compatible cells (the egg chooses which of the hundreds of sperm to let in) at the right time in the menstrual cycle, hitting that 24-hour window for optimal chances of conception *and* successful implantation in a receptive endometrial environment in the womb, is statistically less likely than winning the lottery. All of the preparation ahead of that fateful release is immense. Out of dozens of maturing eggs, there is one (occasionally more) egg that is eventually transported from the ovaries into the fallopian tubes through a poorly understood mechanism which doesn't involve the fallopian tubes actually being attached to the ovaries. If you and your partner are undergoing fertility treatment, this pathway is artificially stimulated and can often result in more than one egg. This means a higher chance of having fraternal twins: around 1 in 5 IVF deliveries in the UK are twins,[1] but this figure is dropping as many clinics now have improved technology and only transfer one egg instead of two or three.

Anyone undergoing fertility treatment is far more familiar with the importance of egg and sperm 'quality', intrinsically linked with our diet and lifestyles. People embark on fertility or reproductive journeys in lots of different ways; some men donate sperm, some women choose to act as surrogates, others freeze their eggs and couples go through the process of creating embryos in vitro (IVF) to improve their chances of becoming parents. Modern medicine has allowed lots of different types of parents to start a family in situations that would not have been possible even fifty years ago. Before embarking on expensive treatment, couples are advised to adopt healthier diets and improve their lifestyle: the obvious ones such as stop smoking and reduce alcohol, reach a healthy weight to support the huge metabolic change that pregnancy entails. A healthy weight for the father (or sperm donor) is also implicated in big changes in risk for psychiatric and neurocognitive disorders; it is no longer just the mother's health that takes centre stage. In fact, the importance of men's health and the health of their sperm has become much more widely understood and discussed, with some major changes taking place to sperm quality and sperm count in the past fifty years that have raised alarm amongst scientists and medical professionals alike. A nutrient deficiency can lead to sperm that aren't well formed or which can't swim well. Smoking and a high BMI can drastically reduce sperm quantity and carry a greater risk of genetic abnormalities, which increase the risk of miscarriage.

For men trying to conceive, a nutritious and varied diet with a focus on physical activity and reducing toxic exposures like alcohol, smoking and plastics is as important as for the mother. Age-related changes are also relevant to men, which is often not recognized because the change is not as drastic as it is with women's age. Nevertheless, the science is clear; men's fertility potential declines with age, and what they eat and their lifestyle directly and independently impact the future health of their offspring. In my own clinical practice, I recommend that if couples are trying to conceive, both parties need to engage in dietary and lifestyle changes.

There are many branded fertility supplements that offer a selection of nutrients associated with improved fertility. The one most of us are aware of, and which has very strong evidence of benefit, is folic acid or folate. The other is iron. Other nutrients including zinc, selenium, coenzyme Q10 and copper have varying degrees of clinical evidence and may be helpful. In fact, fertility and pregnancy is one of the windows of opportunity where I am more inclined to be supportive of supplement use. As you'll learn throughout the rest of this book, it's rare to find convincing evidence that supplementing is useful for other times of life.

For those who have an unplanned pregnancy, these considerations and additional supplement choices might never be made. Especially for a first pregnancy when many younger adults are pleasantly (or not so) surprised at falling pregnant. After all, as many as 60 per cent of pregnancies in the UK are unplanned, though this number is declining as we are generally having less sex. And what does this mean for those successful pregnancies that weren't planned? What of the dozens of women who ask me in hushed tones whether they should worry that they were drinking cocktails in Mykonos before finding out that they were actually pregnant? The good news is, it is often OK. A few drinks are often involved in decreased inhibitions and increased sexual activity at that very specific time of a woman's cycle where hormones are encouraging her to have more sex. To those who generally have a healthful lifestyle, eat nutritious foods and don't smoke, take drugs or drink to excess, the cocktails on the weekend aren't going to have a disastrous impact. One bad note in the entire opera is likely to go unremarked; it's when there are multiple clashes and off tones that we tend to notice.

Top nutrition tips when trying to conceive for men and women

Overall dietary pattern	• The Mediterranean-style diet: high in plants and unsaturated fats; moderate in dairy and fatty fish; low in added sugar and red meat
Plants	• Plants should make up at least half of your plate • Eat a range of colours for a variety of nutrients and polyphenols • Ensure a diverse intake of plants including seeds, nuts, fruits and vegetables • Avoid pesticides where possible • Choose whole fruits instead of juices
Carbohydrates	• Make higher fibre swaps to foods you regularly eat, like switching white rice for pearl barley • Choose whole grains over processed/refined options • Limit sugars and artificial sweeteners in drinks, snacks, baking and cooking, opting for honey as a sweetener where possible • Avoid UPFs

Protein	• Plants can be great sources of proteins packaged up with other nutrients • Limit red meats and processed meats • Some previous research suggested that soy may impact sperm quality, but a recent meta-analysis shows no effect in moderate use.[2] If there is male infertility in the family history, then avoid having a high intake (for example, 3 portions a day)
Fats	• Extra virgin olive oil, plants (for example, nuts, seeds, avocado), and oily fish are great sources of healthy unsaturated fats vital for fertility • Omega-3 is essential; try to have around 2 portions a week of oily fish • Plant-based omega-3 is also useful but additional supplementation may be needed • Limit poor-quality saturated fats, for example, fried food and processed meats • Avoid trans fats which are found in UPFs
Dairy and its substitutes	In women: • Choosing full-fat milk and dairy optimizes fertility • Dairy is a great source of calcium and iodine • Have 1–2 portions a day of fermented dairy, such as kefir and full-fat yoghurt • If you don't drink cow's milk, choose iodine- and calcium-fortified options In men: • Prioritizing full fat is less important

Works in progress

Conception has happened, a successful sperm has fused with a healthy egg and the golden window of opportunity is officially open. The series of steps that take place in the first few days are mind-boggling. From a single fused cell with mixed genetic material from sperm and egg, a transformation begins to a multi-cellular organized mass. Where does the energy for this come from? The building materials? Long before the developing embryo implants and instigates the development of a brand-new complex organ called the placenta, our endometrial lining is secreting a variety of growth factors and nutrients known as 'endometrial milk'. This reaches the rapidly dividing trophoblast (another word for the group of cells that are organizing themselves to become an embryo) and signals the womb to get ready for some major structural changes.

For the first ten weeks, the developing embryo relies on existing supplies from the egg and sperm. This is why having well-nourished egg and sperm is so fundamental to a successful pregnancy. There's some support through the endometrial milk, and then there's the unpredictable magic of successful genetic combinations. There's only a 1 in 5 chance that a fertile couple will get pregnant if they have sex in the best 24-hour window for conception around ovulation. After conception, as many as one in four pregnancies are lost in the first trimester, most likely due to an incompatible genetic combination resulting in an unsuccessful pregnancy.

Despite the biological commonality of miscarriages, and the fact many women won't even know they've had one, they can be heart-breaking. Anyone who has had an early pregnancy scan will remember the sound of the impossibly rapid heart-beat. Anyone who has seen a scan at 10 weeks will tell you that there is so much complexity already visible. The first signs of a head, the beginnings of arms and legs, the buds of fingers and toes. Like a tiny alien waiting to take shape. Then, when the embryo already has a beating heart and the foundations of a nervous system, both of which are heavily reliant on adequate amounts of nutrients such as folate, the baby begins to receive its nutrition directly through the placenta. The placenta is unique as it is an entirely new organ that our body builds to support this new life. The building instructions are contained in the zygote formed by the egg and sperm. Half of the zygote becomes the embryo and later the foetus, whilst the other half becomes the placenta. The blueprint for both new life, and the organ that supports new life, is all decided by the combination of egg and sperm. In fact, recent science suggests that the sperm, and thus *paternal* health, plays a much bigger role in healthy placental formation and function than the egg.

The developmental milestones of the zygote, embryo and foetus are all well understood thanks to developmental biology and the wonders of scans that allow us to observe the developing baby from all angles and in minute detail. It is such an awe-inspiring process, the way the right cells migrate to the right place to form organs at the right time, and even more fascinating is how development adapts when these migrations sometimes get confused. Some babies are born with their hearts facing the wrong way, or organs that are in

FIGURE 5. The stages of foetal development.

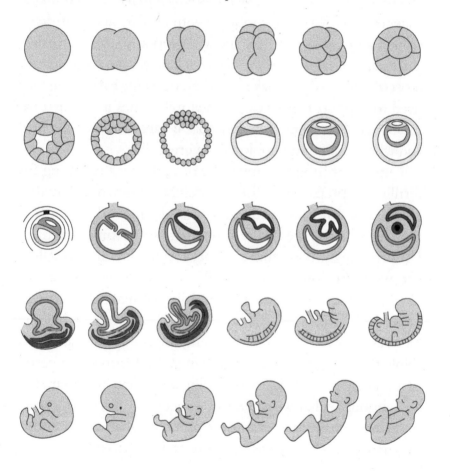

a mirror image configuration. And yet, most of the time, the body adapts and development continues.

An important blocker to a varied and nutritious diet in the first trimester is nausea and sickness, which the majority of women will contend with and some may even need medical intervention for. Hyperemesis Gravidarum (HG) is a very severe form of pregnancy sickness which makes even drinking water difficult. Women who suffer with HG are at risk of dehydration and will usually need medical support to make sure they and their babies stay healthy. So what can women who feel sick most of the day do to make sure they are eating everything they need to support the developmental milestones in the first trimester? This is where pre-conception care becomes essential and where our gut microbiome is a great ally.

Unpopular though it might be now, the idea of eating for fertility in preparation for a potential pregnancy, whether planned or not, is something we should all work towards if there is a chance we might impregnate or become pregnant. Unsurprisingly, diets that support fertility are also excellent for overall health.

This is not to say that improving dietary intake during pregnancy isn't helpful, of course. So if you and your partner are 18 weeks or even 32 weeks pregnant, for example, please don't think it's too late to make some changes. In fact, each trimester of pregnancy brings its own specific nutritional requirements, and although what we eat before conception has a big impact on gamete quality and early development, what we eat during pregnancy also has lots of fundamental roles to play.

The first trimester: introducing womb juice

We've discussed the fact that for most of the first trimester the developing embryo is not actually connected to the placenta, so nutrients are not reaching the rapidly dividing and differentiating cells through the bloodstream as they do later on in pregnancy. A yolk sac forms just two weeks after conception, providing nutrients to the developing embryo and eventually becoming the site where the umbilical cord is attached to the placenta. What's fascinating is the new science around endometrial glands and their role in releasing growth factors and nutrients such as proteins, and even providing necessary immunosuppression to make sure our immune system does not reject the embryo as an 'intruder'.[3]

When you were a tiny bundle of cells in your mother's womb, these endometrial glands were likely responsible for providing what you as an embryo needed for the yolk sac and to continue development, as well as sending the correct signals for growth for the placenta. Many of my clients undergoing fertility treatment know the importance of a good endometrial lining for successful implantation, and it looks as though the lining itself and how well our body is able to deliver nutrients and growth factors to the endometrial glands during the first weeks is crucial.

Nutrition in the first weeks of pregnancy

What does this mean for the mother? She's in the first weeks of pregnancy, the egg and sperm quality have already played their part and placentation with nutrient exchange through the blood isn't going to happen until weeks 10–12. So how do we support women in this time to maintain their best possible nutritional status? The focus is to help maintain good nutrition despite the morning sickness. Eight out of ten women suffer with nausea and vomiting in the first trimester, and the idea of eating complex meals with lots of strong flavours is nauseating in itself. I remember trying to eat some sweetcorn and sweet potato fritters with poached eggs and avocado with my first pregnancy, knowing it would be a nutritious option, and running for the door the minute they arrived. Nausea in pregnancy is no joke! And it lasts the majority of the day for most women.

My advice is to identify the window of time in the day when you are feeling the least sick. In that time window, plan to have a very nutritious meal in smaller portions to allow for reduced appetite. It is one of the times when smoothies can play a really helpful role: served ice cold, smoothies made with nutritious whole foods are usually much easier to deal with when you have nausea. Put together a handful of frozen berries, frozen spinach, an avocado or banana, beetroot, mixed seeds, mixed nuts or a spoonful of nut butter and blend with ice. Colourful vegetables provide helpful plant chemicals that can improve blood flow, fibre for a healthy and helpful microbiome (more on the maternal microbiome later!) and several essential vitamins and minerals.

Another piece of advice is to take foods that you do tolerate and make them as nutritious as possible. When pregnant with my second daughter, I found salt and vinegar crisps to be an absolute miracle cure for my nausea. Of course I could not survive on salt and vinegar crisps alone, so I found some alternatives for those moments when my nausea seemed worse: salt and vinegar seaweed thins, salt and vinegar baked chickpeas and salt and vinegar mixed nuts all became staples in my laptop bag. With my first daughter, I loved cucumber, mint and apple, which was easier to turn into a staple snack of cubed cheese, apple and cucumber to which I sometimes added some red grapes and celery and snacked happily on throughout the day.

The thing about the first trimester is that it often forces you to slow down, which is great as stress and its associated hormones are not helpful, but it can make women feel really exhausted. A balance of eating when possible, making food as nourishing as possible, napping when you can (seriously, twenty minutes before 3 p.m. is all you need) and making sure you incorporate movement throughout your day will help provide the nutrients and optimal blood flow your womb needs at this point. Avoid sitting for hours at a time, restricting blood flow to the pelvic area, and make the most of your favourite way to move with low impact, whether that's walking, swimming, dancing or cycling.

Lastly, a note on miscarriage and abortion. If you do lose your pregnancy or make the hard decision to terminate, know that you are not alone and there are amazing support groups and women you already know who will be able to offer you support. Losing a pregnancy at any stage comprises an emotional and physical loss, and it's really important to give yourself the space and time to heal and to replenish all of the energy that has gone into the initial stages of new life. Eating plenty of nutrient-dense foods high in iron, plant chemicals, fibre and protein, and taking at least three months for your cycle to re-establish, is essential.

Dietary recommendations for pregnancy loss

Nutrient	Description	Food Sources
Protein	Proteins, comprising amino acids, are crucial for cell repair, especially after pregnancy loss. They play a vital role in healing and recovery.	Red meat, poultry, fish/ seafood, eggs, milk/ dairy products, legumes, nuts (for vegetarians).
Fruits and vegetables	Rich in vitamins, minerals and antioxidants, they aid recovery and reduce the risk of recurrent miscarriages. Eating a variety ensures intake of essential nutrients like vitamins C and A, and folate.	Leafy greens (spinach, kale), berries, citrus fruits, cruciferous vegetables (broccoli, cauliflower).

Vitamin E	A potent antioxidant, Vitamin E supports miscarriage recovery by reducing inflammation and promoting tissue healing.	Vegetable oils (olive, sunflower), rice bran, sunflower seeds, almonds, hazelnuts.
Iron	Iron is essential for producing red blood cells, carrying oxygen and maintaining energy levels. It aids in repairing and healing the body, especially after the heavy bleeding that can accompany a miscarriage.	Fortified cereals, grass-fed beef, lentils, spinach, dark chocolate, tofu.
Vitamin C	Supports the body's healing process, reducing inflammation, boosting the immune system and aiding tissue repair and regeneration. Essential during the physical stress of a miscarriage.	Citrus fruits (oranges, grapefruits), berries, kiwi, bell peppers, leafy greens (spinach, kale).
Calcium	Important for bone health, nerve and muscle function and blood clotting. Calcium is crucial for recovery, especially following the nutrient losses of a miscarriage.	Dairy products (milk, cheese, yoghurt), leafy greens (spinach, kale), nuts and seeds, tofu.

Folate	Necessary for tissue repair and new red blood cell formation. It's important to check with a doctor regarding MTHFR* gene testing for folate absorption.	Green leafy vegetables (watercress, Chinese flowering cabbage), mung beans, red kidney beans, dried seaweed (nori).
Magnesium	Reduces inflammation and promotes healthy cell growth, vital for tissue repair after a miscarriage. Also linked to reduced depression risk.	Cocoa powder, pumpkin seeds, nuts (almonds, pine nuts, cashews), quinoa.
Hydration	Essential for overall health and recovery, water helps prevent dehydration and minimizes bleeding risk. It's important to maintain adequate hydration levels.	Aim for at least 2 litres of water per day.

The second trimester: enter the placenta

You've arrived at week 12; if you're in the UK and under NHS care you'll have your first ultrasound scan showing your baby

* The MTHFR gene has been identified as a gene which codes for a protein involved in folate metabolism.

moving around and hopefully growing well. In most other high-income countries in the world you've already had a couple of scans, but this is the point at which pregnancy loss becomes less likely. Only about 3 per cent of pregnancies that make it to week 12 end in miscarriage so many women feel more relaxed, unless they are at higher risk or have suffered a pregnancy loss before. You and the baby are officially sharing nutrients through the placenta, which is an amazing organ. Its complex vascular system is unique, exchanging nutrients and waste products, and permitting gaseous exchange of oxygen and carbon dioxide.

Maternal blood pools around foetal capillaries, allowing the exchange of what's needed and what is no longer useful, to go from mother to baby and back. Everything that is in a mother's

FIGURE 6. The fetoplacental unit.

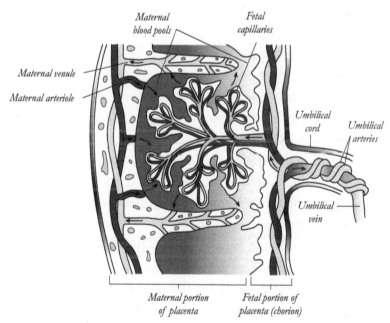

FIGURE 7. A developed human placenta with umbilical cord.

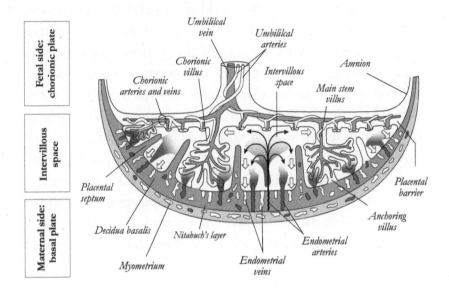

blood will arrive at this interface and be shared with the developing baby. It's easy to see why having a really healthy blood supply and good vascularization (the amount of vessels) is so important. When either is compromised, there are consequences for the baby. A lack of blood supply can result in intra-uterine growth restriction (IUGR) and a slowing of the baby's growth and development. If the vessels themselves are not healthy or there is an issue with increased blood pressure at the placenta, it can result in gestational hypertension, pre-eclampsia and eclampsia, which is a serious medical emergency.

Thankfully, diet can hugely reduce the risk of these pregnancy complications. For pre-eclampsia, a guideline based on the existing literature highlights the importance of a high-fibre diet rich in fruits and vegetables, and low in sugar, salt and fat.

Probiotic fermented foods such as natural yoghurt are also recommended, as they are clearly beneficial for the maternal
microbiome[4] and have a measurable impact on reducing the risk
of pre-eclampsia.

Generally, women in the second trimester feel better and have
more energy, and nausea begins to recede. If this is your first
pregnancy, your uterine wall has never been stretched significantly
so you might have quite a neat bump. Subsequent pregnancies
tend to show earlier because that elasticity has already been tested.
Your appetite and your energy might be back and there are other
changes to your body that might start to show thanks to the
ongoing hormonal changes. This is the trimester of incredibly
rapid development and definition, key milestones in neurological development and an opportunity to make sure all of the
building blocks needed for optimal growth are readily available.

During pregnancy there is a higher protein requirement
than usual. The average adult gets roughly twice the amount
of protein they need from food alone in the UK, Europe and
the US. Believe it or not, protein deficiency is not a thing to
worry about for anyone who eats enough food, though the
protein supplement industry will have us think otherwise.

In pregnancy, high quality protein from food is essential. Protein supplements are generally not advised, as some trials have
shown growth restriction for babies whose mothers increased
their protein intake with supplements. The protein we absorb
from food as part of a varied diet goes towards all the amazing
structures needed to build a baby: the placenta as it continues to
grow with the growing baby, the baby itself, the hormones,
enzymes and neurotransmitters needed. Pregnancy is a high-
protein requirement task for our bodies!

Alongside this protein requirement we also know calcium and iron are really important. Women increase their blood volume by 45 per cent in pregnancy, and many women go into pregnancy unknowingly low in iron. Iron is essential to make healthy red blood cells which then carry all the nutrients, gases and hormones to and from the baby through the placenta. Without enough iron, this process cannot happen optimally. Luckily, many protein sources are also rich in iron: meat, eggs, fish, lentils, nuts and beans are all examples of such foods. Calcium should be eaten in a variety of foods from dairy to calcium-set tofu, leafy greens and tinned sardines or anchovies with the bones still present. Again, many of these foods are also high in protein and some in iron too.

What foods should we avoid in pregnancy?

The issue for most people in countries like the UK is that convenient, UPFs are much easier to find in our food environment than are the products I just mentioned. Cooking from scratch is fairly rare and many women will eat pre-packed or ready foods in pregnancy for convenience and cost. Unfortunately, there is an overwhelming amount of evidence that shows how harmful UPFs and sugary drinks, refined carbohydrates and other pre-packed foods can be to both mother and baby.

The second trimester is a brilliant time to set the right dietary habits for the rest of the pregnancy and beyond. Completely excluding UPFs is virtually impossible, so the 80:20 rule, where 80 per cent of our food is not UPF, is a good one to follow. Reducing the consumption of UPFs and pre-packaged foods as much as possible and using this opportunity to eat whole, nutritious foods really is an investment worth making.

The third trimester: first tastes and preparing for birth

The third trimester is about preparing for birth for the mother, but for the developing baby it's all about first tastes. Most mothers will feel their baby moving in the third trimester and the first interactions start taking place. Babies will respond to touch, sound, temperature changes and even flavours. Chemicals that flavour our food make their way into the amniotic fluid surrounding the baby, which the baby then swallows and tastes with their developing sense of taste. Some fascinating studies have shown that babies exposed to flavours like garlic, spices and broccoli in the womb are more likely to accept these flavours when they begin to eat solid foods.

Studies in twins show that liking garlic has some genetic variability, as does a dislike for coriander! For most tastes and flavours, exposure in the womb (was your mum eating Marmite when pregnant?) and early childhood increases the likelihood that you'll like that food later in life. This makes choosing a variety of healthy foods in pregnancy even more important as tastebud training for later life.

So the fun bit is experimenting with food, enjoying strong flavours if you no longer suffer with nausea and generally using this as an opportunity to train the developing palate to be as widely accepting as possible to lots of different beneficial plants. This is also a time of critical brain development, as the baby learns to hear, starts to see changes in light, tastes the different food Mum is eating and generally becomes more perceptive of its surroundings: the brain is undergoing phenomenal changes. I will go into this later, but I urge pregnant mothers not to drink alcohol. And this advice really persists into the third trimester; often women think the third trimester is less sensitive, and it is for many things, but drinking alcohol risks damaging the developing brain. Alcohol is a carcinogenic neurotoxin which should not be a feature in these particular 40-ish weeks of our life course.

As our bodies prepare for birth, some amazing changes happen. The pelvis has moved and realigned to make birth as easy as possible, and the breasts are often ready to go with some colostrum. This contains bioactive components with immune-enhancing properties: antibodies, lactoferrin, lysozyme, lactoperoxidase, α-lactalbumin, β-lactoglobulin, and fat that carries important vitamins and polyunsaturated fatty acids. It is unique and only present for the first few days following the birth, after which it is replaced by a completely different composition: human breast milk. A note on colostrum is that it can be safely expressed and stored in frozen syringes ahead of the birth in case you need it, but it's not something to stress about. Some women – especially first-time mums – don't have this ready supply of colostrum to harvest in the weeks leading up to the birth, so please don't worry if that is the case for you.

It's a busy time for pregnancy. The mother's body is being stretched to its limit, the baby is growing rapidly and storing subcutaneous (under the skin) fat to help it survive by providing the energy baby needs in the first few days out of the womb. There is still a huge amount of extra blood circulating and excess weight to carry, new breast tissue and a brand-new milk to start producing, and the mother has to prepare for what is essentially a physiological trauma: giving birth.

Birth is absolutely amazing. The first time I gave birth I was so in awe of my body. It made this whole tiny human and then it pushed it out and I walked out of the hospital the next day. I was apprehensive of the unknown quantity of birth but was incredibly lucky to have a relatively quick labour, vaginal birth with only some gas and air, and no perineal tearing. I also had brilliant care on a quiet night in January. September is a much busier month for births (thanks to Christmas/New Year's Eve conceptions) and that might impact how calm and supported your birth might be.

Of course I am fully aware of the wide-ranging experiences women have giving birth. My own second birth experience with my breech emergency Caesarean section was much harder than my first, exacerbated by the fact I was in the middle of my MSc finals and PhD viva (I know, it's a miracle I passed!). It's quite unpredictable, and it's important to remember that it can be dangerous just as much as it can be completely natural. The statistics for birth outcomes vary widely between countries, with the UK falling far behind compared to other European countries,[5] and I often think that's because of the way our birthing facilities are set up and staffed. The staff that work on these wards are absolutely amazing people who have a huge fund of kindness and compassion, but there just aren't enough of them, they aren't paid well enough and they don't get enough days off. Not enough staff, not enough continuity of care and simply not enough time, space and preparation to ensure women can have a positive experience means that the UK (similarly to the US) has very variable birthing experiences and outcomes.

Preparing for birth is very important both mentally and physically. During birth we lose a lot of fluid, undergo a huge shift in physiology from hormones to heart rate and uterine muscle contractions, and we always lose blood. What we eat in the weeks leading up to the birth can help create adequate stores for our body to repair and recover. High-iron, high-protein foods are a priority, and eating enough fruit and vegetables is crucial for our overall nutrient status and to make sure we are feeding the star of the show.

Maternal microbiome

The maternal microbiome spends a lot of its time communicating with the developing baby by sending out chemical messages, known as postbiotics, which directly impact development. It's implicated in healthy placental formation and supports maternal and foetal health by producing even more postbiotics than usual from hormones to necessary vitamins and enzymes, as well as a plethora of amino acids which can be used to help build healthy tissues.

Preparing to colonize the sterile infant gut, the vaginal microbiome undergoes enormous changes leading up to birth. From a standard shield of mostly *Lactobacillus* designed to keep any pathogens out, there is a full-on transformation. The maternal gut microbiome starts populating the vaginal microbiome with strains that resemble the population we see in the mother's gut. Creating a blueprint for the baby's own gut microbiome, this is an astounding and clever way to confer the first steps to a fully functioning immune system as the baby exits into the world.

For this reason, vaginal birth is associated with better health. Children born by Caesarean delivery are more likely to develop asthma, hay fever and the autoimmune conditions coeliac disease and type 1 diabetes.[6] This is likely because that initial seeding of the gut microbiome is an instrumental and key point in the development of a healthy immune system. In fact, our immune system relies on constant communication with the gut microbiome, with 80 per cent of immune system tissue in the gut. By removing the carefully designed maternal microbiome transfer, we essentially miss a step in the evolution of a healthy gut biome.

As I described earlier, my second daughter was born by Caesarean delivery, and we are both alive, well and birth injury-free now thanks to that delivery. Caesareans are a lifesaving medical intervention when needed, and having an increased risk of asthma does not mean you will definitely have asthma as an individual. As we've seen, there are endless opportunities throughout pregnancy, and we'll see that there are many after birth, to make sure we provide all the best building blocks for a healthy and happy life. What is worrying is the increased rates of elective (not medically necessary for physical or mental health reasons) Caesareans. Whilst medically more predictable, they do not offer the same benefits and recovery trajectory as vaginal births. It's an unpopular opinion, but I think it's important that women are properly informed of the risks which Caesareans carry for them and their babies in the short and long term. Too often Caesareans are seen as an equal option to vaginal birth, but this is not the case and I believe we should be doing much more to support women towards an increased likelihood of a successful vaginal delivery.

Exciting research is ongoing to try and close the microbial gap between vaginal birth and Caesarean birth babies. One company, BoobyBiome, has characterized the unique strains found in babies' poo and in mother's milk to try and create an optimal probiotic for those babies who might need an extra hand. Others are researching the practice of 'vaginal seeding'[7] – taking a swab of vaginal fluids from the mother and smearing the baby's face with it after a Caesarean section. The first RCT on this has just been published as I am writing this chapter, and it seems it could be safe and beneficial. So whilst I did not do this with my daughter as its safety and efficacy back then was still unknown, it could become common practice soon.

The good news is, we have another extremely clever mechanism by which our maternal microbiome can continue to support our baby's health and strong immunity, and it's free. It's called breastfeeding.

Birth and breastfeeding

The days and weeks after birth are a tornado of change: recovering from birth and suddenly having a tiny creature completely dependent on you is quite the lifestyle shift. One of the most common misconceptions after birth is that women can't produce enough breast milk for the baby. This can be true for some women, but they are a minority who have physiological or medical reasons why they can't breastfeed. The education on breastfeeding is woeful in the UK and the US, with many healthcare practitioners who work on the wards with women immediately after birth receiving minimal training on supporting breastfeeding.

Meanwhile, formula milk companies gift dozens of units of substitute formula to those same wards, for the exhausted mothers looking for help. The history of formula milk is fascinating and shocking and really deserves a book all of its own, but it's fair to say that I am not a fan. A formula which was originally created to save the lives of those babies who could not access breast milk, designed for survival, has now become an ubiquitous replacement solution to breast milk. On so many levels, this is hugely problematic, but before I explain the benefits and how to support breastfeeding with diet, I want to make clear that I am not anti-choice for parents who can't or don't want to breastfeed. Trust me, I was one of the mothers who was given formula milk when my first baby hadn't gained enough weight, and I have so many stories from women who spent painful hours trying to increase their supply, pumping at two in the morning before going to work at six.

My viewpoint, based on the science and the clear relationships between infant feeding and health, is that all babies should have access to breast milk, whether from a lactating mother OR from donor milk banks. The future holds freeze-dried breast milk from a company in the US, and potentially even microbes engineered to create breast milk components. These should be the obvious alternatives before we consider processed and powdered cow's or goat's milk. I'll go so far as to say that I think it's irresponsible to encourage women to use replacement formula unless it is necessary to do so, and that all parents should be transparently informed of the associated health outcomes beforehand. Of course, some babies will still need replacement formula, and this should remain accessible and affordable.

But the market for infant formulas is growing at an incredible rate, projected to be worth nearly $80 BILLION by 2030. Nearly 20 per cent of global formula consumption is in the United States, and the UK sits at close to 10 per cent.[8] China has seen a huge increase in infant formula use as the first choice from birth. Alongside this huge market in Western Europe and North America, there is a low breastfeeding rate. This is despite the global aim (for child and maternal health outcomes) to reach 70 per cent global breastfeeding rates by 2030. In fact, it's astounding to see how only about 30 per cent of mothers in Western European countries reach *any* breastfeeding at 6 months.[9] For context, the WHO recommends exclusive breastfeeding until 6 months and continued breastfeeding alongside solid food introduction until at least 2 years old.

This is probably a good time to look at the differences between breast milk and formula milk. For the lactating woman, breastfeeding helps speed up recovery from childbirth thanks to its helpful side effect of contracting the uterus back down to usual size. It also lowers the risk of breast and ovarian cancer, strengthens our bones and reduces the risk of osteoporosis, lowers the risk of metabolic diseases such as hypertension and type 2 diabetes and can strengthen the bond with the baby thanks to the oxytocin released as part of the symphony of hormones at play. These associations are all well documented in medical literature and have been for decades. It is part of the reason why breastfeeding is recommended to women for their own health.

For the baby, the benefits are also well documented and

understood. Breast milk offers a complex and adaptive mix of nutrients and immune mediating proteins, live microbes and prebiotic fibres which change at every feed. Morning feed at 2 weeks old in the winter is completely different to an evening feed at 4 months old in the summer. Hormones change, antibodies change, microbes change and even the amount of water changes to provide more hydration in the warmer months. There is instant protection from gastro-intestinal infections which can be fatal, especially in babies born prematurely. It lowers the risk of developing diabetes and obesity in adulthood and provides all the nutrition a baby needs for optimal growth and development, *for free*, without the need for any equipment.

As I mentioned earlier, I used formula milk with my first born. I am not blind to its benefits. It is convenient and easy enough to prepare as long as you have access to clean water, or enough money to buy ready-mixed formula. Anyone can feed the baby, removing the mental and physical burden from the mother, which is huge when you are exhausted and on the brink of ill health from the physical toll of being a new mother. It is measurable, meaning you have a set amount of formula you give your baby per feed, removing the comfort sucking that most babies love to do at the breast. If your baby is not gaining weight as much as your doctor/midwife/health visitor would like, formula is likely to fix it. If your baby is allergic to something in your breast milk from your own diet, hypoallergenic formula can be hugely helpful, avoiding weeks of elimination diets to try and identify the allergen whilst your baby is desperate and in pain.

There are no health benefits of formula for non-allergic

babies that I know of. There are situations in which formula can be an absolute lifesaver for women suffering with their mental health and exhaustion after birth. Can all the benefits of formula be provided with donor breast milk or one of the other solutions in the pipeline? Absolutely. And that is what I hope readers of this book will take away; I am in no way suggesting that full-time breastfeeding is for every mother or an option for every baby. I am asking you to consider that it would be much better to have human milk as the alternative for human babies.

Just as we have successfully increased breastfeeding rates through targeted interventions in countries such as Rwanda (87 per cent), Sweden (62 per cent) and Sri Lanka (82 per cent) to help improve the health of the population, I am certain we can make some effort to improve the UK and the US. The UK is currently the worst in the whole world (only 1 per cent of mothers breastfeed exclusively to 6 months), so the only way is up.[10]

A guideline on nutritional needs whilst breastfeeding

Nutritional needs	Portions (per day)
Energy	Add an extra snack or slightly larger meal portions as you need extra energy!
Protein	2–3 servings of legumes, lean meats, poultry, or fish
Calcium	3 servings of dairy or calcium containing alternatives (for example, calcium-set tofu)

Iron	2 servings of iron-rich foods
Vitamin A	1 cup of carrots (2 large carrots/12 baby carrots) or sweet potatoes (one medium–large potato) and a serving of dairy
Vitamin C	1 orange and 1 cup of strawberries or red peppers
Vitamin D	10–15 minutes of sunlight exposure and foods like salmon, dairy and mushrooms
DHA	2 servings of fatty fish per week
Fibre	5–6 servings of fruits and vegetables, nuts and seeds
Fluids	8–10 glasses of water, plus other fluids like tea and coffee

Introducing the gift of food: complementary weaning basics

Introducing first foods is the most delightful phase. For so many parents, it is a dreaded milestone, filled with fears of choking (a real but mostly avoidable threat), constantly wiping smushed foods (a given), waste, and a collection of expensive contraptions to sit, feed and fully cover baby, to prepare and store foods, and practically remodel your kitchen. When you were a baby, this was the time when you learned so many of your own food preferences which you might still be aware of today.

Working with many mothers and delivering workshops on

infant feeding, I've often been surprised by just how daunting this crucial part of development can be. Anyone who has attended one of these with me knows that my usual recommendations are simple: a simple hand-held blender or NutriBullet is all you need (but a fork will also do), one or two softer tipped spoons are useful for baby to learn and chew on, and you may want to buy a couple of bibs to save little outfits from getting saturated in food. The only item I feel is worth investing money in is a good high chair with variable foot rest and seat height. There are lots of brands that do these now and they offer infants and children the independence to join and leave the table whilst still being at an appropriate height *sitting at the table with the family*.

The problem with many modern Western infant feeding practices, brought on by strict scheduling and the unusual idea that children should eat separately to their family, is that they isolate the infant in their feeding experience. High chairs with their own trays often result in a disjointed mealtime, and one factor many of us hugely underestimate is the importance of teaching our children how to eat food through example. There are hilarious videos on social media showing babies sitting on their mother's lap, hoping that one of the forkfuls of foods flying above their heads is meant for them. Mouth agape, they stretch out their little necks in anticipation, smacking their lips as another mouthful bypasses them for their mother. These videos show us exactly how children learn to recognize and anticipate food, how to chew it and eventually to swallow it.

By placing children in high chairs, covered in full upper-body plastic bibs, and feeding them food whilst facing them without any meal context, we are missing an opportunity to share in the joy of food with them. It is an important part of sensory and behavioural development for children to be able to touch, squish, smush, taste, spit out, splash and, yes, even throw food on the floor. These are all steps children take to learn more about what food is and how to handle it. They look to their caregivers and, later on, their peers to see which foods are safe to try and which aren't. Today we see a growing problem with infant feeding: from first formula feed to first liquidized and pasteurized plastic food pouch, some infants don't get to practise tasting different foods and flavours much.

Do I disagree with the use of pouches for children altogether? No, of course not. They are incredibly useful as a mess-free snack or as a backup food if one of my children gets hungry whilst at the playground. What I do see as an issue, in my clinical practice as well as in the data, is the measurable contribution which UPFs (such as some baby cereals, biscuits and snacks) make to young children's diets. In the UK, children consume nearly two thirds (61 per cent) of their daily energy intake from UPFs[11] – more than in the US and Australia, or anywhere else in the world. What I try to encourage expecting and new parents to do is to see the introduction of food as an opportunity and not a burden. Giving babies first tastes of food as you are cooking, letting them sit on your lap and playing with any safe foods you have on your plate. Having fun with the idea of food, letting them make a bit of a mess, showing them what it's like to eat fresh fruits and vegetables, how to peel a hard-boiled egg and what corn on the cob tastes like.

There are, of course, safety considerations, and understanding the difference between gagging and choking, and the importance of preparing food so it isn't a hazard, as well as knowing which foods to avoid (for example, crunchy crisps and whole olives which can get stuck in small children's throats), is important. Washing and cooking foods thoroughly is worth it to avoid pathogens, and babies shouldn't be left unattended whilst trying foods in the first few months, but within these safe parameters we should let children explore.

One last thing to mention is the importance of introducing allergens (the eight major ones are milk, eggs, fish, shellfish, peanuts, wheat, soybeans and tree nuts). In the 1990s, paediatricians thought that reducing exposure to allergens might reduce the risk of allergies. Pregnant women and nursing mothers were advised to avoid peanuts, shellfish, sesame, gluten and dairy. Some women I've worked with are still advised to avoid these foods today. Much like the flawed advice of putting newborns to sleep on their tummies (which increases the risk of Sudden Infant Death Syndrome, aka SIDs, and was popularized by one doctor in the US), this advice does the opposite of what it was intended to do. Allergy rates shot up, and when microbiome science started to reveal how the infant microbiome informs the baby's immune system on what is and isn't safe in the world, it all made more sense.

Unless the pregnant mother herself is allergic, introducing babies to allergens in the womb, through breast milk and in the initial stages of weaning (i.e., by 9 months old) can significantly reduce the risk of allergies.[12] So eat with your baby, dip your finger in peanut butter, feed them a tiny pinch of soft scrambled eggs and let them taste organic full-fat yoghurt as soon as they are interested (normally no earlier than 17 weeks old). Enjoy the first stages of this new life and serve your baby bitter vegetables like broccoli and nutrient-rich foods like beans and tofu. Most babies will try anything you serve them; the hard bit comes in the toddler years, as we'll cover in the next part of the book.

Expecting common sense: the science of pregnancy

When we look at the evidence for pregnancy and the first 1,000 days, there are a few key points that are rooted in sound evidence and make for great advice. The Mediterranean diet is an effective, universally beneficial dietary pattern that will help to protect the mother's and the baby's health in the short and long term. It will also increase the chances of conception, especially if both parents eat this way. I've boiled it down to: whole grains, legumes, beans, fruits, nuts and vegetables with extra virgin olive oil every day; oily fish, eggs, poultry and fermented dairy products like yoghurt and traditional cheese several times a week; red meat and sweets only occasionally.

Eating ultra-processed foods and sugar sweetened or artificially sweetened drinks is not good for us, especially in pregnancy. Children should be introduced to whole foods, not pre-packaged foods in squeezy pouches. I was shocked to find out that there is an increasing incidence of children with weakened lower jaw muscles because we are reducing the opportunity for them to chew their food. Pureed, super soft UPFs don't help our children to learn how to chew.

It is a skill best learned between 6 and 9 months and it requires a variety of textures. Infants under the age of 2 get as much as 69 per cent of their daily calories from UPFs. This has to stop; we need to do better for our children and vote for politicians who care about making a healthy food environment for future generations a priority.

My final note on pregnancy and what I feel everybody should know going into this stage of life is a critical look at some unpopular topics. Namely, alcohol, caffeine and forever chemicals. I'll keep this one brief because I actually think it's pretty simple, and going into huge detail on the chemistry and epidemiological data is almost reductionist when we consider a few key fundamentals.

As we've seen, the first 1,000 days form a critical path in building a new life. The blueprint of the cells, organs and connecting tissues that make up a human body that will (hopefully) last somewhere close to 100 years are formed in this time. Our sensory processing pathways, our brain structure, the formation and education of our immune system – all happen in this time frame. A 3-year-old's brain is 80 per cent of what it will be in fully fledged adulthood. This specific window in the life course truly is the golden window of opportunity; this level of planning and structural foundations is never repeated again. The way our hypothalamic–pituitary-adrenal axis is wired will predict how stressed we are as adults, how likely we are to suffer with hypertension.

With this in mind, alcohol is a teratogenic, carcinogenic neurotoxin. A teratogen is a substance that causes congenital disorders in a developing embryo or foetus. Alcohol is well known to cause changes in development, including epigenetic changes to key pathways that will then contribute to that future baby's behaviour, facial features and development.[13] Alcohol is a Group 1 carcinogen, which means it is well understood to directly *cause* cancer in humans. Alcohol crosses the placenta, so drinking during pregnancy exposes the developing baby to this risk. Alcohol is also neurotoxic, which means it is well understood to be toxic to neurons – i.e. the cells that make up our brains and nervous systems.

Some interpretations of the available epidemiological data on drinking in pregnancy conclude that it's not that danger-ous and drinking in pregnancy could be OK. I have yet to meet a colleague in public health, paediatrics or medicine more generally who would choose to advise a pregnant woman to drink. When the biological mechanisms underpin-ning the question are so clearly stacked against drinking in pregnancy, picking a couple of epidemiological, cross-sectional studies to show that light to moderate drinking is probably all right seems very short-sighted to me. It's true that most women will reduce or completely stop drinking when pregnant, and it's also true that many women do have the occasional drink and have healthy babies. The problem is, there are too many variables that are unknown. How effective is maternal alcohol clearance? Is the foetus at a par-ticularly sensitive point in development? Is there a genetic susceptibility that is going to be activated due to this expos-ure? How much and how often is the mother drinking? Is the mother taking other medications or recreational drugs? For me, the evidence is clear: if you are having unprotected sex to get pregnant or you are pregnant, don't drink alcohol.

Caffeine is an interesting one, because its effects are less well understood. However, the evidence is very clearly against caffeine consumption in pregnancy.[14] The good news is that a good decaf coffee can deliver the benefits of coffee without the risk which caffeine poses to pregnancy. Sorry to be the bearer of bad news here – I love coffee. But in pregnancy it is not our friend.

Finally, 'forever chemicals' and plastics. A relatively modern phenomenon, we now have plastics and chemicals that stay with us forever in all people. An unborn child will inherit some of these chemicals, such as PFAs and BPAs, directly from its mother. Unfortunately, this area of research is still pretty under-reported, and many if not most people reading this won't have known this is a problem. There is a plethora of research looking at how these plastics and chemicals impact our health. They are implicated in the sharp decline in human fertility rates (1 per cent decline every year, making us 50 per cent less fertile as a species than we were fifty years ago).

The problem with these chemicals and plastics is that they are ubiquitous, so the first thing to learn is how to spot them. The second is to try and reduce them as much as possible, at least in this golden window of the first 1,000 days. To put it simply, reduce the plastic in your life: Tupperware, plates, cups and cutlery, furniture, shower curtains, cling film – where possible remove or replace with natural fibres. Non-stick pans, stain-proof materials, many paints and fire-retardant furnitures contain forever chemicals. The advice here is to replace your pots and pans where possible and try to avoid decorating a house or a nursery with new materials during pregnancy. Every day, open your windows and let fresh air in; these chemicals are absorbed through skin and in the air. Avoid perfumed lotions, personal and home fragrances, shampoos and soaps. I personally use natural oils fragranced with essential oils like jasmine, orange blossom and patchouli. Lastly, use paracetamol sparingly. There is mounting concern about its safety in pregnancy, and my reading of the current evidence suggests we shouldn't be quite so liberal in using it. Great when it's needed, best avoided if not.

Every Body Should Know This

- The first 1,000 days refers to an exact window of time from the day of conception to a child's second birthday. It adds up to 1,000 days (give or take, depending on whether a baby is born prematurely or not).
- Conception and pregnancy are called the Miracle of Life for a reason: it's an absolutely amazing stage where life is brought into being and we should protect it through our food and lifestyle choices.
- What we eat and drink has a direct, measurable impact on our health and our baby's future health.
- Breast milk is better than formulas and should be made accessible for all mothers and their babies.
- Knowledge is power: making choices in specific risks requires us to understand those risks. Alcohol, caffeine and certain man-made chemicals are risky.

- Countries that make early life policies a priority have better health outcomes, productivity and overall life satisfaction. Investing in future generations and their caregivers is always a good idea.
- Our eating habits and preferences are formed from the earliest days.

PART 2

The Rollercoaster Years: Puberty and Adolescence

As we saw in Part 1, once a toddler reaches 2–3 years, the golden window is finished and the majority of brain development has happened. So what happens next? Where are the key points in our children's development? What on earth is going on with puberty and adolescence? A period of life that is woefully underserved by society and by science, children and adolescents are all navigating key stages of life in the hands of parents, the education system, a built environment and a virtual world that has become part of their development in ways my generation could never have imagined. Neurodevelopmental biology, psychology and identity philosophy are outside the scope of this book, but there are some key moments where we can make an impact, and where we should be paying close attention for overall health.

Growth during childhood is steady but nowhere near as steep as it is during infancy or adolescence. The decreased growth rate in toddlers (1–3 years old) and preschool children (3–5-year-olds) is often associated with a reduced appetite and food intake. I have worked with so many parents who come to me when their children are between 2 and 3 years old, worried at just how little their child is eating now compared to when they were 11-month-olds. The truth is, toddlers are naturally going to have reduced food intake, and this is because of the growth curve slowing down. It's also because toddlers start to get a sense of freedom and independence, and food intake is one of the only things they have full autonomy over.

If we place ourselves in a toddler's shoes (or preferably bare feet or barefoot shoes where possible so they can strengthen their proprioception and foot muscles!), we quickly realize that almost everything is decided for them. What they wear, what they eat, activities for the day, nap times, play mates, music, toys, routine, time spent outdoors ... it is almost all out of their control. Giving toddlers agency over some choices (This outfit or that outfit? This book or the other? Playground or library?) can work wonders for cooperation throughout the day. In fact, if we realize that toddlers may refuse to eat at a given time or place, or refuse certain foods, because that is the only choice they are getting in the whole day, it starts to make a little more sense. You may have been a 'fussy eater' as a child for the very same reason. No one likes being left with no choice!

If we couple this new-found independence with reduced appetite, what we get is parents everywhere panicking that their adventurous and generous eater is suddenly eating like a small bird. One of my clients was initially worried that her baby was eating too much. 'He eats portions as big as my own,' she would tell me. Just a few months later she had the opposite problem: 'He barely eats anything at all, I'm really worried about him.' There are of course some children who do need help and who do struggle with eating. Problems with chewing, swallowing, texture intolerance, severe dislike for colourful foods and emotional trauma can all manifest as very disrupted eating that will most likely appear with other issues including weight loss or lack of appropriate growth rate, sleepiness, withdrawal and distress at mealtimes. The earlier these children receive help the better the outcomes, so if you are worried, please get help.

For the majority of cases, the best approach is to be consistent and persistent. As a parent or caregiver, providing a range of nutritious foods at regular times is a big first step. Giving our children the space and freedom to choose what to eat from that selection means we have to respect that they may not want to eat. Forcing them to eat or punishing them for not eating, introducing guilt or shame into mealtimes or giving them one favourite food (milk or formula being the most common culprit) will teach negative associations with food and reduce the chances of the child meeting the minimum dietary diversity needed for optimal growth.

Young children are very sensitive to their hunger and satiety signals. They will ask for food when they are hungry and they will, if you let them, tell you when they are full. They only learn to suppress or override them due to external pressure. I spend a lot of time with my clients helping them to reconnect with their own body's signals, which is such a shame as we are so well attuned to start off with. Some periods of time in childhood bring with them an insatiable hunger. Understanding the human growth curve is a roadmap into that natural response.

Early foods

- **Peanuts**: Contrary to previous advice, introducing peanuts early (around three to six months) can reduce the risk of developing peanut allergies, especially in high-risk kids with allergic parents. Products are available to make this introduction easier.
- **Eggs**: Eggs are a highly nutritious food containing protein, fats, vitamins A, D, B12 and B6, calcium, magnesium, lutein and zeaxanthin. They are often one of the first foods that children learn to cook and are a great option for weaning.
- **Vegetable Soups and Stews**: These can be excellent sources of diverse fibres, polyphenols and complete plant protein combinations. They retain water-soluble nutrients and are a good way to introduce a variety of vegetables.
- **Whole Grains**: Foods like spelt, rye and pearl barley can be included in soups and stews to provide energy and prebiotic fibres.
- **Legumes and Beans**: These are recommended for a healthy diet and can be introduced in the form of hummus or as an ingredient in sauces and stews.
- **Diverse Vegetables**: Offering a variety of vegetables, especially those rich in polyphenols and other nutrients, can help ensure a balanced intake of vitamins and minerals.

- **Fruits**: Whole fruits are generally a healthy addition to a baby's diet, providing essential vitamins and fibre.
- **Full-fat Dairy**: Full-fat natural yoghurt, kefir and cheese are great foods for babies and young children.
- Remember to introduce new foods one at a time and watch for any signs of allergies or intolerances. It's also important to prepare foods in a safe manner for babies, ensuring they are the right texture to prevent choking.

Understanding the human growth curve

In the 1920s, a scientist named Richard Scammon plotted the first human growth curves which have since informed the science of growth in childhood and adolescence. There are four main areas of human development: physical, behavioural, cognitive and emotional. They are all intricately interlinked and affect each other in direct and indirect ways.

We know from harrowing studies of Romanian orphans, discovered in 1990 after the fall of Romania's last Communist dictator, that children who are neglected and deprived of emotional nurturing suffer with terrible cognitive, behavioural and physical consequences.[1] As you might have guessed by now, it is useless to try and separate human beings into discrete themes. Every aspect of our lived experience impacts the next. I believe in nutrition as the uniting tool of

FIGURE 8. Growth rates for different body systems in humans between ages 0 and 20.

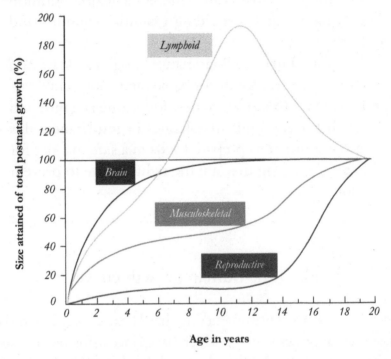

the human experience that can help improve all the areas. For this next part, Scammon's 1920s growth curves help to explain the amazing changes which our bodies undergo in the first two decades of life because, as you can see, there's a lot going on beyond the first two years of life.

The first two years are a rapid, steep incline of growth, where hunger is frequent, food is life and foundations are built. Then there is a slowing of this curve towards more of a plateau, at least for musculoskeletal (muscles and bones) and reproductive organ growth. The brain reaches 80 per cent of complete growth by the age of 3, so in terms of growth, crucial structure is in place pretty early on in childhood. The brain changes in adolescents are to do with the refining and strengthening of synaptic pathways (also known as synaptic pruning), which is an absolutely critical window we will touch on later, but it is not a growth phase. The next steep incline in musculoskeletal and reproductive growth isn't seen until 12–14 years of age and is also known as puberty.

But what about the lymphoid? Many of us are familiar with our lymphatic system because of the glands that can become swollen in our neck when we are sick, for example. Others might know it's important because of lymphatic drainage massages. The truth is, the lymphatic system and the lymphoid organs such as the lymph nodes and vessels that make it up, are underserved by popular science. They play a pivotal role in the maintenance of all our tissues and are an effective front line for our adaptive immune system; that is, the immune system which creates a specific attack against a pathogen. While the innate immune system is one that we have from birth which generally alerts our body to impending danger with generic SOS signals like swelling, the adaptive immune system, which develops with challenges such as infections or vaccination over time, identifies, creates and deploys the best possible weapon against the guilty pathogen with higher efficacy and specificity.

The development of lymphoid organs is absolutely fascinating.[2] Before birth, specialized groups of cells form initial patches of lymphoid tissue in the gut. As we've discussed earlier in this book, the gut plays a fundamental role in immune system function, and the fact that some of the very first lymphoid tissue we grow is in the gut is testament to that. Secondary lymphoid organs such as tonsils, adenoids, those found in tear ducts and in the peritoneum (a pivotal structure that holds our internal organs in place) all form after birth; hence this huge growth curve we see throughout childhood until puberty.

The enteric nervous system is the largest accumulation of nerve cells outside the central nervous system and is embedded in the lining of the gastrointestinal system. When people refer to the gut being like a 'second brain', this is what they mean. The enteric nervous system can operate independently of the central nervous system and there is constant bi-directional communication between this system and our immune system. To add to this, immunity and nutrient intake are synchronized thanks to our body clock, or circadian rhythm. The overall picture is one of careful timing, clever activation and preparing to beat pathogens, but also to prevent disease proliferation from our own cells.[3]

This is interesting, because it is the roadmap to our immune system. The lymphoid tissue and its connected tissues and cells are where our immune cells will gather to decide on battle, clean up rogue T-cells and identify any potentially dangerous cells of our own. This amazing growth of tissue is taking place in our schoolchildren, and we can help to shape the kind of immunity they will have with the lifestyle and diet they are exposed to.

Lymphoid tissue plays a crucial role in regulating inflammation. During development, having too little lymphoid tissue can result in a reduced ability to carry out an appropriate immune response to infection. A severe reduction in lymphoid tissue is known as lymphoid hypoplasia. On the other side of the coin is lymphoid hyperplasia, an increase in lymphoid tissue, which is often seen in response to infection and is the body's way to ramp up the front line. As children go to school, mix with their peers, experience lots of stress and are exposed to lots of different bugs, their lymphoid tissue grows with them at an incredible pace. To support this development, exposing children to natural environments that have soil, plants and fresh air is so important. Making sure they have adequate nutrition to support this tissue growth can make the difference between a robust, fast-acting immune system, or an under-performing system.

In chronic inflammation and diseases such as Crohn's disease, we see the formation of tertiary lymphoid tissue, where the body creates a specific site to try and address the problem. This can happen at a later stage in life and we see it in diseases such as arthritis, but the vast majority of the growth we see is in this period of childhood from 2–12 years old. Any parent will recognize the frequency and relentlessness of the average of nine (up to twelve) different viral infections that children will battle through each school year. The lymphoid tissue grows and adapts with each one like a network of personalized boxing gyms, ready for the next round.

The velocity curve, an example of which you can see below, shows us the sheer speed at which children seem to grow in height every year. You can see for this child, they grew 10 cm in their fourteenth year. That is peak velocity! But they also grew nearly 7 cm at 10 years old, so it's not all about puberty. These rapid growth years bring with them an

FIGURE 9. Velocity curve of growth between ages 7 and 17.

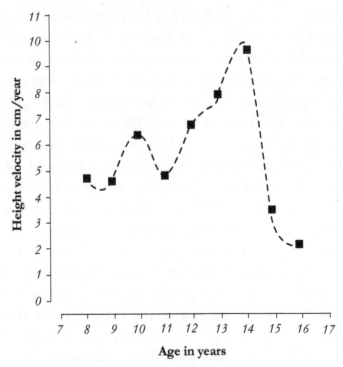

increased need for the building blocks for height: strong bones and muscles.

In children who don't achieve optimal nutrition for growth, their height will become stunted. Stunting is an important concept in child development and nutritional status because it doesn't describe a sudden weight loss due to disease, and it also doesn't describe the height of children because of their genes. Some children are small and some are tall, but a stunted child is one that didn't reach their full potential in growth because of a lack of adequate nutrition.

Stunting is a measure of nutritional status used mostly in

global health and international reports to monitor how children's nutrition is progressing. It is unusual to use stunting in the context of high-income countries as it is typically a result of chronic undernutrition that can stem from maternal undernutrition and persist through childhood. For example, 56 per cent of children in Burundi, 38 per cent of children under 5 in Afghanistan, 16 per cent in Bolivia and almost 2 per cent in Australia are stunted.[4] The UK doesn't report any data on stunting, though a study by Imperial College found that British children are steadily decreasing in stature compared with their European peers, and are now falling behind in growth rates. This worsening of growth trajectories is likely due to a decrease in food quality as well as reduced access to nutritious food due to austerity and cost of living crisis.

Hormones, hormones everywhere

Assuming children do have adequate diets, puberty kicks in around the age of 11 for girls and 13 for boys. Adrenarche is the process by which adrenal glands kick into action, starting the road to pubic hair, increased libido, increased body odour, production of androgens and the making of sex hormones. This fervent activity peaks around the age of 20 and then starts to slow down with age.

Other hormones that play a pivotal role in human growth are human growth hormone (HGH) made in the pituitary gland, insulin released from the pancreas, thyroid hormones from the thyroid glands, glucocorticoids from the adrenal glands, prolactin in the pituitary gland and gonadal steroid hormones which are sex hormones produced in the gonads (ovaries in females and testes in males). It is a concert of different hormones being released from all over the body signalling tissues to grow, store, differentiate and function to help us reach adulthood, when growth will eventually stop by age 18.

Whilst hormone therapy is used in some cases, always under the supervision of a specialist paediatrician, the best way to support adequate hormone production for growth is, you guessed it, an adequately nutritious diet.

Key nutrient deficiencies in young women living in the UK.[5]

- **Fibre:** over 90 per cent of adults do not meet recommended fibre intake.
- **Iron:** 48 per cent of women of reproductive age (18–50 years) consume inadequate iron.
- **Folate:** only 2 per cent of women aged 18–35 years meet the recommended folate requirement to lower the chance of having a baby with a neural tube defect (600ug/day).
- **Vitamin D:** a large proportion of women and men have inadequate vitamin D intakes and are mainly getting their vitamin D from sunlight.

My top nutrient-dense foods for women and adolescents

1. **Eggs:** A good source of iron, containing all essential micronutrients apart from vitamin C.
2. **Mushrooms:** Contain a wide range of micronutrients, including essential B vitamins and vitamin D, which strengthen the immune system and could even reduce cancer risk.
3. **Nuts and seeds:** An excellent source of polyphenols, fibre and omega-3 fatty acids, to improve your gut microbiome.
4. **Wholegrains:** Naturally high in fibre with a range of vitamins and minerals.
5. **Leafy greens:** High in polyphenols, micronutrients and soluble fibre.

For the above, it's important to note that the definition of 'adequate intake' is debatable. Recommended Dietary Allowances (RDAs) are the levels of nutrients that, on the basis of current evidence, are deemed by the Food and Nutrition Board to be adequate to meet nutritional needs. We should always remember that everyone is unique when it comes to nutrition.

The brain on steroids

Earlier in the book I talked about the 'synaptic pruning' that takes place in adolescence. There is a big, important change in brain structure and function that takes place for teenagers, and they are very rarely supported or understood through it with adequate emotional or nutritional support. I find this particularly ironic as it is also the age at which we expect young people to perform exceptionally well academically in order to secure their desired career trajectory.

It's actually a cruel coincidence that our education system is set up with exams as the end goal. Just as our brains are trying to refine and define what the most useful neural pathways are with the potential for creativity at a high, we are demanding that teens cram as much information as possible to succeed in exams. This is all in the context of peer pressure, increased stress and cortisol flooding the brain, exceptionally high androgenic activity and a terrible diet. Teenagers consume the smallest amount of fruit and vegetables, the highest amount of UPFs, the least diversity of whole grains, beans and legumes and are most likely to take up drinking/smoking/vaping or recreational drugs at this time.

Why have our tweens and teens come to be the most forgotten group? Like the elderly, they are often perceived as burdensome and difficult to manage, and are often left to their own devices, which increasingly means their various screens nowadays. Where bored teenagers in the 1970s and '80s would steal bikes and spend days causing a different kind of mischief, bored teenagers today disappear in a world of social media. Online bullying and virtual lives through hyper realistic games can quite literally result in sitting still in the same position for hours whilst causing a perceived stress response without any of the physical activity to help dissipate some of that stress.

I have two young children at the time of writing this book and I can already see the pull which technology has on them. I am not one of those parents who has managed to remain screen free, nor do I necessarily believe screens are always terrible. The science on this topic is growing, and there are several groups of researchers trying to quantify the effects of screen time on developing minds. A systematic review of lots of studies[6] concluded that prolonged and frequent screen time is associated with a tendency to seek short-term gratification, which when considering the social exposures a lot of teens experience at this time (sex, drugs and reduced sense of danger) can make for a powerful combination.

Colleagues at Imperial College London are conducting the SCAMP study of cognition, adolescents and mobile phones,[7] one of the biggest studies of its kind. Their findings confirm what most of us probably instinctively know. More than three hours of mobile phone use per day is associated with higher BMI (so a higher risk of becoming overweight or obese) and sleep problems, which are closely linked to behavioural difficulties. The final areas of the brain to develop in adolescence are the frontal and temporal lobes – both of which affect emotions, language and memory processing.

The other issue with the mobile phone and online world is the pervasiveness of adverts that children are exposed to. Adverts for fast food chains, energy drinks and UPFs are presented to them multiple times a day every single day. Repeated exposure to these adverts causes a change in behaviour and food choice; we know this from well-conducted social experiments that see groups of teenagers that don't know each other individually choosing the exact same dish of triple fried chicken nuggets from a list of over thirty food items. The experiment finishes with the teens being shown how many times they were exposed to that food item on their journey over to the restaurant; on their social media feed, on posters in the street, advertised in the taxi and overheard on the radio. The teens had not picked up any of the adverts consciously, but subconsciously it was so well delivered that they all chose the same dish when faced with the option.

The food environment our teens are growing up in is far from ideal for their health and for this last crucial stage of brain development. Applying pressure to governments, schools and corporations like FIFA who still allow fast-food companies to be the main sponsors at sporting events is certainly part of the solution. The persistence of takeaway and convenience food adverts shown during televised events is also astonishing; at times it feels like you're watching pizza takeaway adverts more than the primetime TV show you actually tuned in for. Bite Back 2030 is an activist group founded and run by young people, for young people, to achieve healthy, nutritious foods being available for all. They are doing an admirable job, but they need adults to really get behind this cause and make healthy food accessibility a priority.

Denmark, Finland, Iceland, Norway and Sweden have taken firm moves to monitor the advertising of junk food to children. France actively discourages parents from feeding their kids UPFs and Italy has one of the lowest percentages of UPFs in the world at only 14 per cent of daily calorie intake. Teens need whole food as they are still in a critical window. They need a strong immune system through a healthy functioning gut microbiome; their brains demand adequate building blocks and omega-3 fatty acids to reach their full potential for cognition and for mental health. For girls, the need for adequate nutrition is even more critical in this window of opportunity. Their bodies begin creating and dismantling tissue roughly every 28 days, responding to fluctuating hormone levels that instruct their bodies to build an endometrial lining in their womb, prepare their breast tissue to grow in case of pregnancy, undergo an inflammatory process to release an egg and then lose all of that blood and excess tissue at the start of a new cycle.

Nutrient recommendations and advice

Nutrient	Daily Recommendations	General Advice
Protein	2–3 servings of lean meats, poultry, or fish (75g/3 oz each)	Include lean meats, poultry, fish, beans and nuts
Calcium	4 servings of dairy (250ml/1 cup milk/yoghurt or 40g/1.5 oz cheese)	Consume dairy, fortified plant milks, greens, almonds
Iron	2–3 servings of iron-rich foods (75g/3 oz red meat or 200g/1 cup cereal)	Red meat, poultry, fish, beans, fortified grains
Vitamin A	1 serving of carrots/sweet potatoes & 1–2 servings of dairy	Found in dairy, greens, orange vegetables

Vitamin C	1 orange and 1 bell pepper or 200g/1 cup strawberries	Citrus fruits, strawberries, bell peppers
Vitamin D	10–15 mins of sunlight or 2 servings of fortified foods	Sunlight, fatty fish, fortified foods
Fibre	5–6 servings of whole grains, fruits and vegetables	Whole grains, fruits, vegetables, nuts, seeds
Fluids	8–10 glasses of water per day	Hydration is key; water is the best source

Enter the menstrual cycle

I will never forget my first period. Miserable and feeling grumpy, I woke up and started getting ready for school. I was 11-ish and was in no way prepared for the whole situation but clearly remember a feeling of general sluggishness. My mum took the knickers I had clumsily thrown across the room to pop them in the wash and looked as shocked as I did mortified. A quick introduction to sanitary towels and I was off to school, learning on the fly. Things have moved forwards in leaps and bounds since I was that age – period positivity and moving away from adverts using blue water on sanitary pads is a positive step. Talking openly about our cycles and what periods can feel like has been helped by social media, and I'm much more aware of speaking openly to my daughters about it. What's next for science and research is a better understanding of the physiological needs women undergo throughout their cycle. Published research papers on nutrition through the menstrual cycle are still few and far between, but change is afoot and there are some basics that everybody should know.

Menarche is the term used to describe the first menstruation marking the first menstrual cycle. It is the beginning of a female's reproductive years and it marks a real change in nutritional needs for years to come. The age of menarche is influenced by lots of factors including genetics, exposure to endocrine-disrupting chemicals (known as EDCs),[8] body weight, body fat and how sedentary we are.[9] On average, girls now get their first period earlier than their mothers did. This earlier age of menarche is associated with a 50 per cent higher risk of gestational diabetes (GDM)[10] after adjusting for other factors known to increase risk of GDM.

A varied diet with plenty of healthy whole foods and an active lifestyle is more likely to result in an ideal window of age for the first period (the menarche). Girls are more involved in organized sports now than thirty years ago, but it's sadly still not safe to send young women for a walk or a run on their own, as 97 per cent of women in the UK report being victims of sexual harassment by the time they reach their twenties.[11] Finding a way to make movement and exercise safe for girls is important, and being aware of it as an issue is the first step.

Once girls start menstruating, their bodies undergo a cycle of repletion and depletion as just described, with the building

97

and loss of their endometrial lining. This comes at a cost to the body that has to be fulfilled with good nutrition. The most common nutrient deficiency in the world is iron deficiency, and the more severe iron deficiency anaemia, found in women of reproductive age (15–49) and children. Global estimates show little or no improvement on global rates,[12] which vary widely from nearly 80 per cent in Yemen to 7 per cent in the US,[13] with a global average of 30 per cent.

Heavy menstrual bleeds are closely correlated with iron deficiency[14] which can cause a variety of symptoms including reduced cognitive function, fatigue, exhaustion, brain fog, muscle weakness and dizziness. It's easy to see how this would seriously disrupt schooling and exam performance, as well as quality of life. Iron supplements do work and are effective but they aren't the long-term solution for the vast majority of girls and women. A diet that provides enough nourishment and specifically iron-rich foods is the best way to prevent and recover from iron deficiency. In countries such as Yemen, where food is scarce and getting enough to eat at all is incredibly difficult, it is a humanitarian crisis. But in Europe, the UK and other countries where food is widely available and where we provide an excess of calories per person we need to feed (roughly 4,000 calories are available per person per day in the US), the issue is clearly one of food quality, not quantity.

My hope is that we start nurturing our children and teenagers with whole food again. There are clear windows of growth, change and intense brain development that go on to shape who they become as people and how they enjoy their formative years. The majority of mental health conditions present themselves in this crucial window: 50 per cent of all mental illness is established by age 14, and 75 per cent is established by the age of 24.[15] There are many factors that contribute to mental well-being – it is not all about food – but food is something we can change ourselves and, on average, our kids are not eating well enough for their well-being.

Every Body Should Know This

- How children and teens eat impacts their health now and their risk of disease as adults.
- Children and young people's bodies and food habits are continuously developing. Their nutritional needs are plastic and require us to provide a variety of nutritious foods.
- They need our help to improve their food environment to achieve good mental and physical health.
- Technology shouldn't replace time spent moving and socializing in real life, especially for children and young people.
- Iron deficiency anaemia is one of the biggest deficiencies we see. Adequate nutrition for females who are menstruating is critical to support health, happiness and the last phases of development into adulthood.
- Young men have a much increased need for zinc for healthy testosterone production and omega-3 for brain and hormonal health. Seafood and seeds offer both!

PART 3

The Circles of Life: Adulting

As teenagers, many of us look forward to the freedom of adulthood: the endless possibilities to do whatever we want, eat, sleep and live however we please. The truth is more complex than that, and Eleanor Roosevelt's quote that 'with freedom comes responsibility' is pretty spot on. For many of us who make it into adulthood relatively healthy, these are the years of invincibility: party until three in the morning, sleep for a few hours and somehow bounce back on our feet to go to a lecture/job/next ward round and do an OK job at it.

For some young adults, this is when disordered eating will become a prevalent issue. Hospital admissions for eating disorders have increased by 84 per cent in the past five years,[1] a staggering increase which has caused the Royal College of Psychiatrists to launch new guidelines to help professionals identify and help treat those at risk earlier. Disordered eating and eating disorders are associated with mental distress and trauma; they are not a nutrition problem and should not be treated by a nutritionist alone. The result is malnutrition, but it's critical to always involve a qualified psychiatrist or specialist psychologist in the diagnosis and treatment plan.

It's important to note that many modern diet 'trends' can be problematic for disordered eating. Clean eating, orthorexia (excessive exercise with very prescriptive food consumption) and other forms of restrictive dieting all play a role on the spectrum of eating disorders and many people can experience a range of these issues over their lifetime. Sensory processing and neurodiverse conditions can also lead to very restricted diets and a difficult relationship with food.

Malnutrition is a term used to capture both undernutrition *and* overnutrition, and the most modern form of the double-edged sword is food overconsumption with micronutrient deficiencies. This type of malnutrition is characteristic of industrialized UPFs which are both calorie dense and nutrient poor. Micronutrients such as vitamins, minerals, iron and plant chemicals are usually lacking in UPFs, as is fibre, whilst they are usually abundant in sugar, fat and so-called cosmetic additives that make food look, smell and taste better than it should. This means that when we talk about malnutrition, we are including people who consume an excess of calories but are not nutritionally replete. This is the fastest growing form of malnutrition; a situation in which children and adults alike are consuming more food and more energy than they need, are more likely to experience overweight, obesity and type 2 diabetes, yet are low or even deficient in essential nutrients like iron and folate. How bizarre is that? We have too much poor quality food available in our food environment that leaves most of us overweight *and* undernourished.

Here is the perfect opportunity to bust the myth that nutrient deficiencies are due to our crops and vegetables losing nutrients. They aren't. It is the intense farming practices and industrial processing of fruits and vegetables, trying to extrude the vitamins for juices or to add to foods, that is decreasing nutrient value. In other words, overly processing plants is the issue.[2] I agree that soil health and reducing the use of pesticides and herbicides is critical for our long-term and planetary health, but the reason we are seeing an increase in this paradoxical malnutrition is because we eat mostly foods that are eaten out of a packet, ready to eat, and are *not* crops and plants. The pastries, ready meals, snacks, biscuits, chocolate bars, breakfast cereals, fizzy sweet drinks and white breads with very long shelf lives are the ones that contribute a high number of calories for very little nourishment. The majority of us (90 per cent or more in the UK and US) don't reach the recommended daily requirement for fibre, fruit and vegetables in our daily diet and end up more likely to suffer with obesity, as well as being micronutrient deficient.[3]

Let's get it on

Statistically, early adulthood is the time when most of us typically have the most sex. Interestingly, our rate of reproduction is diminishing in all age groups and young people are generally not having as much sex as expected. Our populations are declining and we are heading towards extinction according to some of the most pessimistic projections. An eternal optimist, I like to think that it's a good time for us to get involved in our own future as a species and, if we want to have children, be aware of the factors that improve or decrease our chances of successful procreation. For those who don't want to procreate, it's worth knowing that all the things which increase reproductive potential will improve your health. Evolution, being the clever biological process that it is, is finely tuned to make sure reproduction takes place when the odds of successful reproduction are pretty high, even though our lives no longer revolve around the core biological priority to procreate and continue our species' survival.

The health of our sperm and our eggs is an accumulation of inherited factors and the exposures over the roughly 90 days of maturation. The thickness and blood supply to our endometrial lining, the crucial bedding for a fertilized egg to land on and implant, depends on stress, hormones, nutritional status and level of physical activity. It is a combination of many factors that work together to try and enhance the chances of reproductive success, and not just one thing that tips the balance. So what does science tell us is the best way to support our reproductive potential? And how can we work to maintain it into later life, when many of us are choosing to have children?

As usual, it's useful to understand the fundamental science that drives the processes involved. At a very basic level, reproduction is about making sure we pass on our genetic information for future generations with bonus points for new genetic mixes that result in more resilient individuals. There's some absolutely fascinating research on how we choose our sexual partners; it's neither as simple nor as cerebral as we think. One of the factors I find most interesting is how our sense of smell plays a part. Pheromones get a lot of air time for their love potion properties, and some perfume companies have made a fortune selling perfumes that mimic these magical, subconsciously sexy signals. They play a crucial role in helping us understand whether we should run or stick around when faced with a potential mate.

What's less well understood is exactly where these pheromones are secreted from. The general consensus is that we excrete them via our skin glands, breath and maybe bodily fluids. There is some suggestion that our gut and skin microbiome are having an effect too, and this makes sense. Our immune system is critical in finding a mate and sustaining a healthy pregnancy. This is because immune compatibility is a really important factor in fertility. The most common example of when this can go wrong is when a rhesus negative female (negative blood types like myself) have babies with rhesus positive males (the vast majority – 80 per cent plus – of the population). In simple terms, if this incompatibility of blood types was not addressed, my maternal immune system might have fought and destroyed my developing babies as it would have identified them as a 'non-self', positive blood type presence.

Luckily it's easy to screen for the 'rhesus' (and worth knowing your blood type!) and if there is a mismatch of negative mother and positive father, we have a simple injection that stops this immune reaction from taking place. I have, however, come across a couple of women in my clinical practice who had suffered recurrent early pregnancy loss, and had not had this simple test done.

So back to the smell of your chosen mate, their skin microbiome, the immune system and gut microbiome, who are all absolute best buddies. The gut microbiome helps to regulate and modulate the immune system, sending signals to the rest of the body on what is happening. It also communicates with the skin biome, translocating some of its bugs to the skin surface and giving out signals including our smell. On top of this, the skin biome metabolizes skin gland excretions, influencing the smell of our sweat. I have now started to think of our smell as the equivalent of microbiome smoke signals, giving anyone in the vicinity a quick update on what's going on inside.

This becomes even more interesting when we consider the impact which our hormones have on our biome and vice versa. In women, there is a term for the oestrogen-loving bacteria: the estrobolome. These guys thrive when our oestrogen is high and produce metabolites including an enzyme which helps to recycle oestrogen from receptors back into the circulation. We know that the gut microbiome and its health is closely linked to the vaginal microbiome and its health, which both influence fertility. In lots of ways, our immune system and gut microbiome work together to try and help us select the best possible match when our sex(y) hormones are highest to try and improve the chances of reproductive success.

Anyone reading this book who is or at some point has been in their late teens and early twenties knows what it feels like to have ragingly high hormone levels. For these young adults, the smoke signals are basically smoke clouds – our microbes and hormones are at full throttle scoping out the potential mates surrounding us. We are at peak reproductive capacity between the ages of 20–25, where we are more than 80 per cent likely to conceive if we are having unprotected sex over the course of a year. This value drops significantly by age 30, and falls to about 50 per cent by age 40.

Each cycle, there are only six or seven days that we are actually likely to conceive. So if we think of falling pregnant as a bit like rolling dice, you need to get lucky with the time of your cycle, known as your fertile window, as well as get lucky with your likelihood according to your age. For men, fertility starts decreasing after 35 and there is a gentle downhill to about 75, but as discussed earlier, diet and lifestyle can massively impact the likelihood of sperm being effective at their job.

For women, the pregnancy rate per month falls to less than 5 per cent after 40. Fertility discussions can be daunting and even as I'm writing this, I feel a bit emotional about it. I'm 36 now so firmly in the rapid decline of potential success cycle by cycle, which is no surprise at all to me but I feel it and its emotional weight. Partly because of my clients going through their own fertility journeys and all the women I have known who have struggled and been through the trenches of fertility treatment, and partly because I would love to have a few more years to maybe experience another pregnancy and another child.

There is more nuance than that, of course, as I already have two children; my chances of conception are actually higher than a woman my age who has not had any children yet. And the other massive factor that we have not mentioned here is the role of the sperm. Men produce millions of sperm – between 40 and 180 million per millilitre. That means that with each ejaculation, there are about 80 to 300 million sperm ready to go, and typically only one of these will succeed in fertilizing an egg. My male clients have managed to significantly increase their sperm quality, sperm count and improve DNA fragmentation

FIGURE 10. Chances of clinical pregnancy depending on day of ovulatory cycle by age.

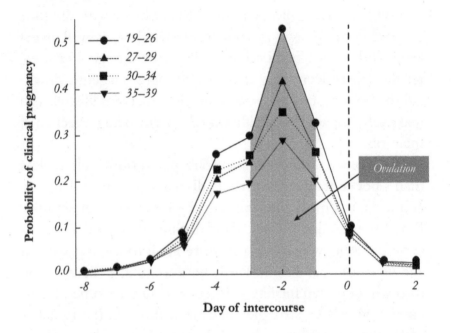

metrics (i.e. less DNA damage) after a few weeks of following advice aimed at improving their health and fertility.

One healthy egg, roughly 200 million sperm in a good ejaculation, a probability of 0.3 if one has sex at the exact right day about 2 days before ovulation and a perfectly primed endometrium to nourish the fertilized egg. You start to see why this whole thing is called the miracle of life. The odds of you being you, that one sperm and that one egg successfully colliding and developing into an immunologically compatible human are really small. Dr Ali Binazir made headlines[4] when he calculated that the odds of each of us being alive from the chances of your parents meeting to the exact genetic combinations that make you you, are 1 in 10^2,685,000, which is basically 0. We are all unimaginably unique.

So let's go back to the role of the father. Often underestimated and underappreciated, male sperm quality does make a big difference. Male fertility begins to decline at the age of 35,[5] and is the biggest factor in successful pregnancy when performing intra-uterine insemination. This might come as a bit of a shock; men rarely consider their own age as a limiting factor to reproductive success and women are often the main focus in the social narrative around fertility, conception and pregnancy. It's women who feel the burden of responsibility to be aware of our biological limitation to reproduce but it truly does take two to tango.

The Developmental Origins of Health and Disease (DOHaD) is the working hypothesis that foetal programming in the womb plays a huge role in predicting the health and disease of the future adult. It is a fascinating area of medical research and one of the reasons why I am so interested in the first 1,000 days of life as the 'Golden Window' of opportunity to prevent disease and maximize health. Paternal programming as a feature of DOHaD is gaining lots of momentum and has given some very interesting insights.[6] Paternal health including smoking status, BMI, stress levels, diet, age and exposure to endocrine-disrupting chemicals (EDCs) all play a role in sperm and seminal plasma (semen) health. These factors have been linked not only to fertility but also to the health of the placenta, the likelihood of neurocognitive and developmental changes and the risk of other diseases. The semen isn't just acting as a transporter for the sperm; it contains active components that directly influence the womb environment and help to modulate gene expression. What the father is doing in the weeks before conception matters just as much as the mother.

One of the things that all my fertility clients mention to me, is their amazement at the emphasis that there is on preventing pregnancy. The way we are taught about sex and fertility growing up is focused on avoiding pregnancy at all costs, as though the chances are inevitably high for ever. It would potentially be more useful to teach young people that the chances are high when they're young, and educate them about the role of the menstrual cycle on fertility. It's also important to highlight the role of the sperm, and how effective sperm can be if given the chance (and why so many babies result from the early withdrawal as a method of contraception which does not have good efficacy!). This is especially relevant for heterosexual and cisgender people, but it's important to have this knowledge for any person who thinks they might want to have children in the future, however they choose to build that family.

I realize that this whole section aligns with my own personal experiences and viewpoint as a female who wanted to have a family from a fairly young age. My goal is to provide the basic context and science for what is a complex and often complicated journey for many.

IVF and other assisted reproductive technologies (ART) are a world of their own with huge amounts of variability in how patients are treated, how their eggs, embryos and sperm are handled, the price points, the success rates and the aftercare. Each country differs widely in how people are able to access these technologies, if at all, and what the probability of success is. Genetic screening is hardly used in the UK, whereas it is almost commonplace in the US. Companies are starting to offer egg freezing as a work package incentive and the narrative that pregnancy in our forties is fairly straightforward has permeated more widely with celebrities such as Beyoncé and Sienna Miller, Halle Berry, Madonna and Uma Thurman all sporting beautiful bumps. Understanding the likelihood of becoming pregnant at different stages in our lives, and the chances of a successful pregnancy with egg freezing and the physical, mental, emotional and often financial toll which fertility medicine can have is really important.

And for those who don't want to get pregnant, know that our hormones and microbiomes make us most sexually active and attractive in peak fertility windows. The most effective form of contraception is abstinence, especially in the fertile window, and understanding which contraception method works best for you is very important in the most fertile years. I was part of the generation of girls who was put on hormonal contraception the moment I considered having a sexual partner. It worked for me. I was lucky to have a mother who helped me advocate for the right level of hormones that matched my baseline biological levels, so I felt empowered to ask for my specific prescription and suffered very few, if any, side effects.

For my own daughters, I'm not sure what the best approach will be when they reach that age. What I do know is that I have relished understanding my own menstrual cycle and working with that knowledge to plan my family and fertility journey. I have already started teaching them about menstrual cycles at a very basic level and hope that that will help them understand their bodies better than I did at an earlier age.

What to consider when trying to conceive

Fertility testing	If you're unsure about fertility health, it's a great idea to get tested. I recommend: - Women: HERTILITY (hertilityhealth.com) - Men: MyMojo (mymojo.ai)
Body weight	Maintain a healthy weight to optimize fertility for both men and women: • Low body fat for women reduces oestrogen and can cause ovulation problems • Low body weight in men can impact sperm quality • Higher body weights, particularly around your middle, impacts fertility in both men and women • Obesity can also put you at much higher risk of problems during and after pregnancy

Lifestyle	• Avoiding alcohol is best in women and men trying to conceive
	• Continue physical activity
	• Good sleep practice is important for sex drive, sex hormones, and maintaining a healthy weight
	• Smoking:
	  ◦ reduces quality and quantity of sperm, which can risk foetal development
	  ◦ In women it can decrease chances of getting pregnant by up to 40 per cent by reducing mature egg collection, disrupting hormone levels, and preventing normal transport of the egg through the oviduct

Taking a toll

Whether trying for a family, trying to avoid pregnancy or having a young family, this whole reproduction window is quite exhausting. Recovering from fertility treatment or pregnancy and birth or the societal pressure of parenthood is all quite a lot. I see many women who come to me five, ten or even fifteen years after having their children and are looking for help to rebuild themselves. Just like fertility, this period of exhaustion is an easy target for marketing and products in general. There are supplements, courses, books, retreats and many other available tools on the market for people who feel 'tired all the time'. I recently saw a meme that read 'I looked up all of my symptoms and Google said I have kids. It's kids, I have kids,' which is quite funny, but also points to a bit of an issue.

The UK and the US do not fare well in various measures of family policies and outcomes. One of these is support for young families, and specifically for mothers who want to work. It is cripplingly expensive to return to work after having a child since there is no free childcare provision until the age of 3. Three years out of the job market at what is a potentially optimal window for professional growth for many women is a long time. Yet there is zero subsidy for private childcare available, and you can only get the thirty hours (which, by the way, is hardly full-time) of free childcare if both you and your partner (if you have one) have a job.

That's a lot of caveats, and those who don't have a job have already endured statutory maternity pay. Directly from the government website:

> Statutory Maternity Pay (SMP) is paid for up to 39 weeks.
> You get: 90% of your average weekly earnings (before tax)
> for the first 6 weeks. £172.48 or 90% of your average weekly
> earnings (whichever is lower) for the next 33 weeks.[7]

I cannot imagine how £172.48 per week, in a city where the
average rent is now £2,000 pcm and a country where it is £1,261
pcm as of August 2023, is supposed to scratch the surface of
food, shelter and comfort for a baby and their parent.

This financial stress applies to anyone undergoing fertility
treatment too, where the cost can be around £5,000 per cycle
and people often spend large amounts of money on supplements, alternative therapies and specialists to bolster their
chances. For those choosing not to have children, or who
cannot have them, they likely have a financial and professional career advantage.

But I digress. Aside from the financial slog of raising children in the UK, there is the physical and mental depletion.
Physically, fertility treatment, pregnancy and birth have a huge
impact on the mother. The changes in hormone levels that
occur are the largest fluctuations a female will ever experience
in her life. The best way we can support ourselves through
this mammoth challenge and change is to prepare well. At the
moment, very little is done to support women who are of
reproductive age and might be considering becoming pregnant. Medical professionals often limit their advice to 'take
folic acid', and with nearly half of pregnancies worldwide
reported as 'unplanned'[8,9] we need to take a more proactive
approach to improving women's health, full stop.

Anaemia is still a leading micronutrient deficiency in

women, which is hugely problematic in maintaining a healthy pregnancy and in preventing complications at birth. Giving birth generally involves losing blood, whether it's a complicated birth or not, so having sufficient iron stores can make a huge difference for recovery and even survival. As our diets move further away from nutrient-dense whole foods and towards UPFs that lack essential nutrients, we are blindly walking into a serious problem not only for the current generations, but also those to come.

Mentally, the modern family unit is problematic for happy child raising. Many parents live many miles or entire oceans apart from family, grandparents and other support networks. The majority of households have an uneven distribution of domestic and childcare labour, leaving women mostly responsible for a huge amount of unpaid work, often in conjunction with the need for paid work. High stress levels and reduced sleep are both very metabolically demanding, so eating well and nourishing our bodies to help mitigate these unfavourable exposures (to put it mildly) is crucial.

It is also important to find your own village before you have a family. Find your people, or prepare financially to hire them, because it is quite tricky to pull a team together when you are just about pulling yourself together after giving birth. I am always very emphatic when I am asked for advice by people preparing for pregnancy: get help in place before the baby comes. I wish someone had told me the same before my first; I'm sure I would have had a much easier time of those first six months if I had. Afterwards, everyone shares their experiences of sleepless, lonely nights and there's a remarkable camaraderie amongst those who support each other. Again, my thought is that being prepared is a good approach to take.

I had very little idea of how intense the postnatal period was going to be. I spent a lot of my pregnancy worrying about the birth, which actually went very well and lasted a relatively short amount of time. Days after giving birth, on my own most days because I didn't know to put help in place and my husband was busy getting our home ready to move into (another strangely popular theme), I was so taken with trying to master breastfeeding and generally keep my baby alive and happy that I virtually forgot to eat or drink anything myself. I ended up back at my maternity unit with the shakes and heart palpitations, feeling faint and very ill. They ran a bunch of tests and essentially told me I needed to look after myself better. It can easily happen, and I went into it very well nourished, healthy and relatively knowledgeable.

One last point on recovering and looking after ourselves is about spacing pregnancies. There is plenty of evidence that having at least 18 months between birth and subsequent *conception* is better for the mother's and the babies' health. Emotionally and physically, birth spacing is actually very important. If you can, give yourself some time to recover between pregnancies, and give your children time to emotionally adjust. The good news is that having children lengthens women's life spans despite the blood loss, hormone rollercoasters and nutrient depletion, and breastfeeding reduces the risk of breast cancer. In fact, being a parent increases life quality and longevity.

Maximum power

Between the ages of 25–35, men and women are at their peak capacity to be in top physical condition. What I mean by that is that we are faster, stronger, leaner, more resilient, more fertile and generally able to achieve more physical feats in this time. Interestingly, we are actually happiest later in life, but this decade is when we can make the most of our physical prowess to nourish and build a body that will carry us into our nineties.

This idea that we can hugely improve our long-term health by nurturing good habits around our thirties is one that is definitely gaining momentum. Preventative medicine is where the majority of healthcare practitioners and healthcare systems aspire to be contributing. Of course the reality is that it is taking a very long time to shift the focus from treating to prevention, but there are some positive trends in younger generations that seem to be a symptom of this understanding. People in their twenties are much less likely to smoke or drink alcohol compared to their predecessors. Weight and strength training are much more mainstream for men and women, and most people know that exercise is important for good health.

What are the best ways to make the most of this magical decade when changing body composition is much easier and you can build a solid foundation of good lean muscle mass to see you through the tougher decades? It's as simple as using your body in as many ways as possible, lifting weights, moving a lot every day, challenging yourself however you can and eating food to nourish that movement. This does not mean protein shakes and bars and focusing on chicken breast every day; it means eating a wide variety of foods in their whole form as much as possible and not counting macronutrients or calories.

A lot of people are so resilient in this window of their lives that they take very little care of themselves: drinking alcohol excessively, sleeping erratically, eating too little or too much takeaway and convenience foods, smoking, vaping and taking recreational drugs in a way that doesn't give their bodies much time to rest. Anyone who knew me in my early twenties will know that I am guilty of taking my resilience for granted. I worked and studied very hard but also refused to miss out on opportunities to socialize and very often slept far too little, driving home at night to sleep for five hours before heading back to university for a full day of lectures. I used to joke that I would sleep when I'm old, but now I know much better.

Luckily for the present and future me, I have always enjoyed exercise and find movement throughout the day is a key driver of my productivity and mental health. I am no athlete, but I am conscious of the fact that I need to maintain my health if I want to make the most of the longevity genes that run in my family. A body fat between 25–30 per cent, with lean muscle mass as a general goal is a good start. My vision for my nineties is to be full of life and laughter, sporting a purple or pink rinse and still moving about independently with my children and (possibly) grandchildren in my life. Having lived with three of my four grandparents in their final days, I have seen how cruel it can be not to be able to get yourself out of bed or to pour yourself a glass of water. They were all sprightly, clear minded, spirited and mobile until the end (all in their eighties and nineties) and I hope to do the same.

Key takeaways for health and happiness

- **Nutrition**: Focus on a balanced diet rich in vegetables, lean proteins, healthy fats and whole grains. Limit UPFs and added sugars, and increase fibre.
- **Exercise regularly**: Include a combination of cardiovascular exercise, strength training and flexibility workouts to maintain muscle mass and cardiovascular health.
- **Quality sleep**: Aim for 7–9 hours of good quality sleep each night. Establish a consistent sleep schedule and create a restful sleeping environment.
- **Stress management**: Implement stress-reduction techniques like mindfulness, meditation, yoga or deep breathing exercises to mitigate the impacts of chronic stress.
- **Regular health check-ups**: Undergo regular health screenings and blood tests to monitor vital health markers, including cholesterol levels, blood pressure and blood sugar levels.
- **Mental health**: Give attention to mental well-being. Engage in activities that promote positivity and consider professional help.
- **Avoid harmful habits**: Stay away from smoking, limit alcohol consumption, and avoid recreational drug use to prevent long-term health issues.
- **Time-restricted eating**: Explore intermittent fasting or time-restricted eating as a strategy for

weight management and improving metabolic health. Simply follow the same 10-hour eating window on most days.

- **Hydration**: Water plays a key role in various bodily functions, including digestion and detoxification. Make sure you drink when you're thirsty and eat plenty of fresh fruits and vegetables.
- **Active lifestyle**: Incorporate physical activity into daily life beyond exercise routines, such as walking, using stairs, or opting for standing desks.
- **Cognitive health**: Engage in brain-stimulating activities like reading, learning new skills, or solving puzzles to keep the brain sharp.
- **Social connections**: Maintain strong social and community ties, as social interaction is a critical component of overall well-being.
- **Environmental awareness**: Be conscious of environmental factors like air and water quality, and make choices that reduce exposure to toxins.
- **Personal growth and learning**: Commit to personal development and lifelong learning to keep the mind active and engaged.

Postnatal perimenopause

A note on an interesting phenomenon which is happening more now thanks to our shifting demography and trend of having children in our thirties instead of our twenties. Many women I work with come to me with postnatal symptoms:

consistent and persistent weight changes, hair loss, skin issues, irregular periods, sleep disturbances, loss of libido, anxiety, rage and loss of motivation. Birthing a tiny human and terrible sleep coupled with recovery from birth and an astonishing rollercoaster of hormone changes will do that to you, and it's a shared human experience for most mothers. Except, some of the women I see gave birth a few years ago. Their symptoms have persisted, changed and maybe evolved into something else. Some say the postnatal recovery period can last many years, but most agree that once the baby reaches 3 years of age, you are mostly back to baseline albeit a little older, wiser and more sleep deprived.

The gap between postnatal recovery and perimenopause is narrowing and I think there is more overlap than lots of us appreciate. My clients having IVF, preparing for pregnancy or egg freezing in their forties report familiar symptoms of night sweats, anxiety, rage, mood disruptions, hot flushes, hair changes, weight changes and a sense of lack of self-recognition. As we keep pushing the boundaries of parenthood, giving people the opportunity to build families later in life when there is often more emotional and financial stability, it's important to remember that our biology hasn't had time to evolve to our new timelines.

Supporting postpartum recovery includes many of the principles already discussed in this book, and hormone changes and recovery are dependent on how we feed our children. Exclusive, responsive breastfeeding brings a period of low oestrogen and no ovulation, whereas women who don't breastfeed return to ovulating more quickly. Breast-feeding also brings floods of oxytocin which is a lovely

FIGURE 11. Changes in progesterone and oestrogen before and after childbirth.

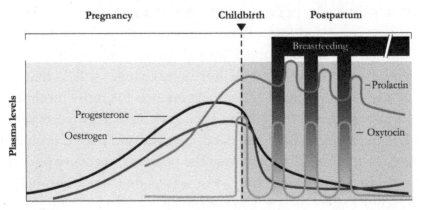

hormone that acts as a neurotransmitter in the brain to essentially supercharge our caring and bonding response.

The graph above shows you how progesterone and oestrogen decline rapidly after childbirth. Earlier in the chapter we saw that oestrogen levels in women peak by the mid-twenties and decline by 50 per cent by the time we are 50. It's easy to see that a mother who gives birth in her late thirties or forties is unlikely to return to premenopausal levels after this period of change, and so our postnatal care should adapt to the individual woman's life stage.

Whether your postpartum period and your perimenopause overlap, or not, it's worth taking note of how you feel in your postpartum period because your progesterone and oestrogen levels fall to a very similar level at both change points. After all my pregnancies, my hair has changed quite dramatically, prompting my husband to ask me if I was OK after he walked in on me brushing several clumps of hair off my head. I also know that, as a usually very level-headed and conflict-avoidant person, I am prone to bouts of rage. I am

sure there'll be some surprises in store for me and my menopause transition, but knowing and understanding my own
reaction to hormonal changes has made so much difference
in my ability to communicate my needs and feelings at different times. Encouraging young women to track their cycle,
note how they feel and learn to recognize when hormones
may be changing their usual behaviour is so important.

When boys become men

Men undergo a seismic shift in their forties that, unlike wom-
en's health, has less of a blossoming societal movement
surrounding it. Unfortunately, the number one cause of
death for men in this age bracket is suicide, and it's called the
silent killer for a reason. Mental health needs have soared in
the past decade, and whilst women present to NHS services
for therapy and treatment more frequently than men, the
rate of suicide is three times higher in men than it is in
women. There are lots of factors that contribute to mental ill
health, including ethnicity, socio-economic status, education,
adverse childhood events (ACEs) and social isolation.

A lack of friendship and support networks can have a huge
impact on mental ill health, and men today are much more likely
to report they have no friends they can call on in times of need
than ever before. Whilst this book is primarily about the impact
of nutrition on our health, it's critical to consider the impact of
mental health and human connection throughout our lives. For
men in their forties, friendship might just be one of the biggest
investments they can make for their lifelong health.

Not only does having friendship and a support network help to prevent serious outcomes like suicide, it also helps to reduce stress and the impact which cortisol (the stress hormone) has on our bodies. Men are disproportionately impacted by increased stress levels when compared to premenopausal women. This is because oestrogen is protective against some of the stress response effects. Cortisol itself increases inflammation and drives metabolic changes that make us more prone to storing fat around our organs and our midriff.

Men are much more likely to use drugs of abuse like cocaine and heroin, as well as drinking alcohol to excess. Evidence suggests that whilst sexual assault on women is still higher, there has been a bigger increase for men, and men are much less likely to report the abuse or seek help following assault.[10] The combination of external stressors like the cost of living crisis, internal unresolved trauma, societal pressure to carry on as usual and a lack of support networks is likely driving a mental health and addiction crisis in men today.

Men's health is undeniably impacted by the rising burden of mental health problems, so for men, it's crucial to think about the following:

- Learn tools to respond to stress positively: breathwork, yoga, meditation and playing music are examples.
- Connect with like-minded people and share your experiences and worries.
- Consider therapy to resolve any past trauma; it's always worthwhile.

- Spend some time outdoors every week; disconnect from work and other pressures.
- Reduce alcohol and avoid the use of harmful drugs like cocaine and heroin.

What happens next?

Like me, you've hit 35 and you're looking ahead at the next fifteen years. Statistically, if you are female you're about to peak in your career; if you're male you have some way to go and you're likely on a rapid incline. You might have a young family or maybe you're planning one, or maybe you aren't at all. Technically, you've reached and passed your peak physical condition. Twenty-one-year-olds start looking really young, barely adults, and you start to act and sound like your parents, surprising yourself and possibly appreciating them more.

In terms of nutrition and health, this is a really variable time. A detailed analysis of over 1,000,000 patient records[11] concluded that though chronic age-related 'lifestyle' diseases had increased in all age groups between 2005–2014 (with the exception of COPD or chronic obstructive pulmonary disease), the relative prevalence of chronic diseases in people aged 35–50 was significantly lower than older age groups. This is the age where you are more likely to die of suicide or a car crash than you are of a stroke. This seems obvious as the diseases listed are age related so obviously increase with age, but it highlights an important point: dyslipidemia (an unhealthy blood fat profile) and hypertension (high blood pressure) are the ones that have significant numbers attached to them, even at these younger ages (7.4 per cent and 11.6 per cent respectively) whilst cancer, type 2 diabetes and stroke all sit between 0.5 per cent and 2.1 per cent. Dyslipedemia and hypertension both sit on the disease pathway to heart disease, stroke and other metabolic diseases, and they are mostly preventable and reversible with lifestyle and dietary changes. These are the first signs of some of the cogs not working at their best.

For women, this fifteen-year window is critical because of the menopause transition. Hormone levels start to change both drastically *and* erratically, contributing to a wide range of symptoms ranging from sleep disturbances to dry, itchy skin, weight gain, severe anxiety and hot flushes. The perimenopause is different for every woman, and I recommend women start preparing for these changes from the age of 35. Globally, women are going through the menopause later in life, from an average age of 48.4 years to 49.9 years,[12] but there is a counterintuitive rise in the rate of premature menopause (before age 40) which is increasing in some populations, from 1 per cent up to around 2.8 per cent of women.[13]

The science on menopause, health and diet is in its infancy in some ways, as the revolution on women's health and research is finally making an impact, but we definitely have enough information to know some key factors in maintaining good health through this change and beyond. After all, the perimenopause can last a few years but our post-menopausal years are potentially half of our life span, if not more. A bit like worrying about birth without planning for the years following it, focusing entirely on the menopause without looking ahead to the rest of our lives is not setting us up for success.

The majority of women will suffer with some symptoms,

some very severe, and some bothersome but not disruptive. The beauty of what we do understand is that it's actually fairly simple to help our bodies through this change, though not necessarily easy.

Top tips for optimizing health in the menopause

- **Eat more plants.** It is amazing how effective simply having more whole plants is found to be in reducing the risk of the most unpleasant symptoms of menopause. Regardless of whether you are overweight, taking HRT or at what age you enter perimenopause, eating more plants works.
- **Aim for a healthy body weight.** Having a higher BMI is associated with worse symptoms and a higher risk of postmenopausal health issues such as womb and breast cancers, type 2 diabetes and obesity. This is easier to achieve pre-menopause.
- **Build and maintain more muscle for an optimal body composition.** This is the time to focus on our biggest metabolically active organ: our musculoskeletal system. Skeletal muscle is a huge organ in our body that secretes myokines, acting like a huge endocrine (hormonal) organ that helps keep us healthy. Using your muscles often will also help maintain a healthy metabolism and is important for mental health and sleep.
- **Cut down on alcohol.** The negative effects of alcohol seem to multiply several-fold for

menopausal women. Whichever way you look at the numbers, it all points to reduction as key. If you still want to drink, epidemiological evidence suggests that 2–3 glasses of red wine per week spread over 2–3 days is a good place to land.

Every Body Should Know This

- Your sexual partner roulette is at least partly influenced by your microbes. They help you choose your partner through chemical messages like smell. Nourish them well with plenty of whole foods and fibre.
- The odds of a successful pregnancy decrease from the age of 24 onwards for females, 35 onwards for males.
- Paternal health, age and the quality of sperm *and* semen play a hugely important role, equivalent to maternal health.
- Building up good body composition with plenty of lean mass and healthier subcutaneous (under the skin) fat mass in your thirties and forties is a good insurance policy for your eighties and nineties.
- Eating and exercising well in perimenopause is worth it. We now spend roughly half of our lives as postmenopausal women.

PART 4

Avoiding the Twilight Zone: Building Your Health Span

I can't help singing Bon Jovi's 'Livin' on a Prayer' in my head when I think about reaching 50 and midlife in general. It's such a catchy song, definitely not written about midlife, but it conveys this message that you're actually only halfway through and also that you've already made it halfway there! What a joy to have reached this specific point in life, where you have already been through so much but still have so much to look ahead to. This time of life is known as the midpoint or midlife, but I've also heard it referred to as the twilight zone and even 'sniper alley', which is quite terrifying. The reason for these names is that often this is the age when more people in our lives start to die. Not from car accidents or from awful early onset cancers, but from diet-related diseases of ageing. Preventable things like heart attacks, type 2 diabetes and strokes, 80 per cent of which could be prevented with diet and lifestyle changes.[1]

The majority of us reading this book can statistically expect to live into our nineties and there will be a fair few centenarians. The late Queen Elizabeth II was sending thousands of letters to centenarians by the end of her reign; King George

V sent a handful of them by bike in 1917 – that's a big increase in 100th birthday congratulations. So what happens at the age of 50? And what do we really need to think about to make the second half of our lives something to look forward to?

As I touched on in the previous chapter, differences in health risks really start to emerge between the ages of 50–65. This is extremely individual, of course, and we all know stories of people who suffered with very poor health earlier, or those who embarked on an amazing health and fitness transformation later in life. The beauty of understanding the variability and factors that influence these changes is that health and disease are not set in stone. For the most part our genes, with a few rare exceptions, aren't precise agents of disease or health. They are part of the musical notes on the music sheet of an entire concerto that is our lives. How loudly, softly, quickly or poignantly the notes are played depends on many other factors including the annotations (epigenetics), the conductor (lifestyle and diet) and who is in your orchestra (microbiome), as well as the hall you're playing it in (the body and context you live in). There's a big difference between me playing Beethoven's 'Für Elise' aged 14 in the school hall, and the London Philharmonic Orchestra doing the same at the Royal Albert Hall. The notes on the music sheet (genes) are the same, but the end product is very different.

What's also important to remember here is that we can't always influence all the factors that go into this concert. It's hard to control where you're born, what parents you're born to, how they will raise you and whether you have access to the beneficial components of a healthy diet and nurturing environment. Inequality in health is intrinsically linked to inequality in resources. Poverty leads to poorer health, and a society which doesn't close the gap on socio-economic divide is also not solving health inequality. These differences in health become very evident in the second half of life.

The Great Equalizer

Women are generally less likely to die than men, until they hit the menopause. The average age for menopause in the US and UK is 51, so it sits beautifully as the starting line for the second half, and it is such an interesting physiological and metabolic change. A pre-menopausal woman is better protected from cardiovascular disease, bone disease and dementia, and has a better overall immune response to pathogens compared to a man the same age.[2] Man flu is, in fact, rooted in some evidence. Oestrogen plays a main character energy role in all of this, gifting us with a natural biological advantage in so many ways, but we have to learn to work with our menstrual cycle. As we've discussed, periods are physiologically and emotionally costly, especially if you have heavy periods that leave you at much higher risk for anaemia, suffer with fibroids or endometriosis which cause immensely painful periods, or struggle with mental health conditions such as premenstrual dysphoric disorder (PMDD) that require treatment and therapy.

Suddenly, women and men are catapulted to a pretty even keel. Women still tend to be diagnosed with cardiovascular disease later than men, thanks to the protective effects of their pre-menopausal years, but they end up suffering with just as many of these diseases after menopause. The ZOE Menopause study[3] showed for the first time that postmenopausal women had worse metabolic responses, measured by blood glucose and blood fat levels, and a completely different gut microbiome fingerprint compared to their pre-menopausal counterparts of the same age. This difference goes beyond ageing and is understood to be due to the menopause itself as a huge shift in a woman's entire biology.

Part of the work I love doing the most is working with women to maintain their natural biological advantage. I relish the fact that, if we can successfully enter the second half holding the reins of these changes, we have a whole lot of life ahead that isn't governed by monthly hormonal rollercoasters and the risk of bleeding to the point of anaemia. I say all of this as someone who considers myself quite lucky. My cycles don't

FIGURE 12. Percentage of the population with heart disease by age group.

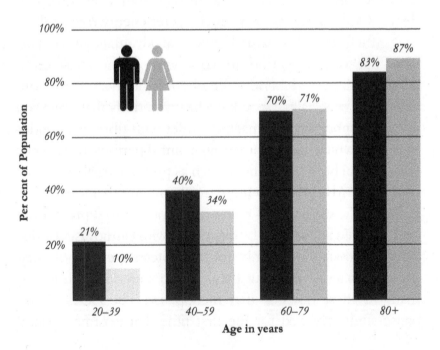

usually halt my life, though after having children I started to suffer with hormonal migraines which, if not caught in time with the right cocktail of interventions, can leave me unable to tolerate any light or do much at all other than lie down in a dark room.

Hormonal migraines

Hormonal migraines are triggered by hormonal changes, rather than the other common triggers such as stress, lack of sleep or caffeine. Menstrual migraines tend to start just before or during a woman's period when levels of oestrogen drop substantially, and levels of both female hormones (oestrogen and progesterone) hit their lowest point. Other types of hormonal migraines can occur at other times of hormonal change, such as in pregnancy, when on hormonal contraceptives, or whilst on HRT for the menopause. Women are three times more likely to suffer from migraines than men, and these hormonal changes are a key cause.[4]

There are a host of options for women to deal with their menopausal symptoms, from combined HRT to knowing more about vaginal lubricants and using testosterone; I think we'll be seeing a lot of personalization in this area of medicine. I can imagine that there might be a way of predicting the symptoms you are most likely to suffer from based on your experiences with your cycles and any pregnancies you've had, in order to best prepare women for the changes and prescribe appropriate medication if needed.

The evolutionary significance of menopause is something I find absolutely fascinating. Present in just a few species, menopause in humans is believed to be functional, preventing women from bearing children at the same time as their daughters do, known as the 'grandmother hypothesis'.[5] This developmental phase, though challenging, is essential. It demands adjustments, just like adolescence, but it is not merely a symbol of ageing. Instead, it should be perceived as a beneficial transformation that has implications for a woman's health and vitality in her later years, as well as supporting and benefiting the well-being of society's children and grandchildren.

It is also the perfect time to re-evaluate and concentrate on nutrition. The foods that work really well for us in our pre-menopausal lives are going to have a totally different impact on our perimenopausal and postmenopausal bodies. The exact same meal eaten the same way in different decades of your life will have a different impact. This is obvious when you think about it (my usual diet during my undergraduate degree was enough to power me through a marathon today), but it is still one of the most common complaints I hear from my female clients. *I am eating exactly the same foods, and exercising more than I used to, but my body keeps changing.*

What I've learned through research in this area and through working with my clients is that the hardest thing to do is accept this change. Not recognizing yourself in your clothes, in the mirror and in how you perceive others now view you is incredibly difficult. I haven't lived through it yet and can only compare it to how alien my own body felt to me in the weeks after giving birth, but for some of the women I work with it is devastating. Embracing that this is a whole new body, with a different biology, is the first step. Understanding that finding new ways to operate this new body at optimal level might take months, when the change can feel so sudden, is the second step. There is no silver bullet. HRT doesn't work for everyone, and HRT alone is never the sole solution. Understanding change and embracing its inevitability is at the heart of making the journey easier – which is also the philosophy at the heart of this book. Unfortunately for women, the menopause is the journey equivalent of white water rafting off a cliff edge; and lifestyle, diet and a positive mindset make for excellent equipment to withstand the ride.

In the meantime, I am excited to be working on some brilliant science with the ZOE team to better understand what the menopause can teach us about optimizing women's health. Harnessing the super powers of our body's health signals, we can learn to predict an upcoming problem. Like an effective radar for a plane, we can see trouble ahead and shift our trajectory much earlier on in order to reduce the risk of collision. The future of personalized nutrition, medicine and health is rooted in this predictive principle, and the advent of community science powered by technology means it is becoming a reality already. One of my first ever studies as an undergraduate[6] looked at how useful mobile phone tests could be to measure cognitive performance when people were drinking alcohol. Before iPhones and apps were commonplace, we used text messages, and honestly the whole thing seems prehistoric now because of the rate of change. It is such an exciting time for science – I could never have imagined then the amount and quality of data we can collect now, from thousands of people.

Historically, clinical and other intervention trials were performed in a few hundred men, mostly white, mostly in their thirties, with no pre-existing disease. From these trials, the effects of pharmaceuticals, psychotherapy, dietary interventions, screening and all manner of health tools were extrapolated to other people: women, people of different ages, people of different ethnicities and people with multiple health concerns. As technology has evolved and our appreciation of the power of personalization has grown, our ability to expand this much further is finally here. The power of prediction lies in numbers, and at last we can start to make this a reality that involves everybody.

The andropause: what to expect and how to mitigate the changes

The andropause is used to describe men's equivalent of the menopause, where age-related changes in hormone levels (mainly testosterone, an androgen or male hormone) can occur. Andropause is a more debated concept than menopause because of the difference in physiology: men experience very gradual hormonal changes, compared to 100 per cent of women who experience sudden changes.[7] Menopause and andropause aren't directly comparable, but it's true that the hormonal changes men face are real and do trigger symptoms which can drastically impact quality of life. These include low mood, decreased sex drive, poor concentration and loss of muscle mass as well as general change in body shape and composition. These symptoms often start gradually, as testosterone declines slowly by around 1–2 per cent each year from the age of around 30–40, and some men never experience the effects of these changes.[8]

Most of the treatment options for this include lifestyle changes, stress management, sleep hygiene and talking therapies, though I've noticed testosterone and even growth hormone therapy being used by some of my male clients who don't like the changes they are experiencing. Hormone replacement therapy (HRT) might be advisable in some cases and can be prescribed by GPs, but is a lot less commonly used than in women.

For my male clients, I do recommend that they look after their overall health and this age-related change by tackling two main pillars: sleep and stress. Men are less protected from the negative effects of stress and lack of sleep, which both have a huge impact on metabolic health[9] and risk of heart disease, high blood pressure and increased fat mass. Correctly addressing sleep and stress together with dietary changes and a focus on good quality nutrition has a huge impact on men's mental and physical well-being.

Tips on foods in the menopause and andropause

Food Type	Tips
Fruits and vegetables	• High volume: these should be at least half of your plate • Aim to eat the rainbow to ensure diverse range of polyphenols • Try to get 30 different plants a week (including seeds, nuts, etc.) • Enjoy in season, frozen, or tinned • Test out fermented foods like kimchi and sauerkraut

Nuts and seeds	• A great way to add variety to your diet • Aim for a handful every day • Store seeds in a jar and add to meals and cooking
Meats and plant proteins	• Use plant proteins, which also tend to be naturally packaged with other beneficial components like polyphenols • Animal proteins can be part of a balanced diet, but limit processed meats and aim to have some meat-free days
Breads, cereals and other carbohydrates	• Aim for higher-fibre choices • Choose options with less added sugars, sweeteners and chemicals • Minimize UPFs which in general have less fibre and more sugar or chemicals
Dairy	• Eat in moderation to gain the benefits (like protein, probiotics and calcium) • Pick less processed options, like natural yoghurt, to avoid added chemicals, preservatives, sugar and sweeteners • Choose fermented options like kefir to support your microbiome
Sweet treats	• Dark chocolate can be a great choice, offering a boost of polyphenols and fibre – pick options with fewer ingredients and a higher percentage of cocoa (70 per cent+) • Fruit, nuts, yoghurt, home-made cakes and honey can be a great choice to enjoy at the end of a meal

Inflammation and stress

The body's natural mechanism of inflammation acts as a defence response against threats or injuries. When someone sustains an injury such as a cut, the body's immediate response is to increase blood flow to the injured area, transporting platelets, white blood cells and defence chemicals to combat potential invaders. Concurrently, the increased blood flow allows swift removal of waste products. This process manifests externally as redness, pain, and swelling – classic symptoms of inflammation. This response occurs on a smaller scale continuously throughout the body to protect us from disease and neutralize harmful by-products of our daily metabolic activity. In essence, inflammation is a beneficial process, but issues arise when it becomes chronic or imbalanced.

Such imbalances might be due to autoimmune diseases where the body's immune system mistakenly attacks our own cells. Chronic, or long-term, inflammation can also result from persistent infections like tuberculosis or from repeated acute (short-term) inflammatory responses that the body cannot correct. This chronic state of inflammation has been associated with various debilitating and life-threatening ailments, including heart disease, type 2 diabetes, mental health disorders, Alzheimer's, and some forms of cancer.[10,11]

Diseases, infection and injury aren't the only causes of inflammation. Modern lifestyles cause low-grade, chronic inflammation which has been labelled the silent killer of the modern world. Activities – or lack thereof – such as sleep deprivation, enduring stress, sedentary habits and dietary choices can exacerbate inflammation. For instance, sleep studies have shown that lack of adequate sleep can stimulate chronic inflammation. Interestingly, the metabolism of the food we consume plays a crucial role in how it affects inflammation.[12] Consuming foods results in an increase in circulating blood sugar and fat, initiating a chain reaction resembling 'mini fires' of short-term inflammatory peaks. Over time, these sporadic bursts of inflammation can establish a chronic state.

Lifestyle changes to decrease inflammation

Body composition	• Remember that weight itself doesn't indicate your body composition (i.e. how much fat and lean muscle you have) – so don't fixate on weight alone • Aim to optimize and stabilize your body composition by optimizing physical activity and nutrition
Nutrition	In general, the nutrition advice I've promoted throughout this book minimizes inflammation, in particular: • Eat a diverse range of colourful plants, rich in fibre • Limit refined carbohydrates like white breads, pastries and sweets • Avoid UPFs where possible • Minimize red meats and processed meats • Enjoy fermented foods like natural yoghurt, kefir and sauerkraut

Physical activity	• Integrate physical activity into your daily life to decrease inflammation • Aim for at least 30 minutes a day of activity (this includes a brisk walk to work!) • See my 10 top tips for integrating activity into your daily routine (Page 171)
Sleep hygiene	• Try to keep a regular sleep routine • Limit technology before bed • Avoid eating after 9 p.m.[13] • Limit caffeine or avoid completely after 2 p.m. • Exercise during the day
Stress	• Practise stress management techniques including breathwork and journalling • Try CBT methods – these can be self-guided through books[14] • Do a course of evidence-based mindfulness[15] • Seek medical support if needed
Alcohol	• Limit or avoid completely • If you do drink alcohol, choose red wine
Smoking and vaping	• Avoid completely

However, all hope is not lost. Our diets offer a key opportunity to reduce inflammation. Certain nutrients can counteract these inflammatory responses. Polyphenols, for example, found in extra virgin olive oil and colourful fruits and vegetables, can help mitigate inflammation. A meta-analysis of studies comparing the effects of lower polyphenol refined olive oil with high polyphenol extra virgin olive oil found that while both caused a rise in blood fats, the polyphenols in the latter significantly reduced inflammation and oxidative stress, showcasing the protective qualities of specific dietary components.[16] Other high polyphenol foods, like garlic, ginger, berries, nuts and seeds, have also shown anti-inflammatory properties, whilst UPFs have the opposite effect. However, rather than focusing on isolated foods, it's essential to consider our overall dietary patterns.

The human gut microbiome, consisting of trillions of unique microbes, plays a fundamental role in regulating inflammation, our health and metabolism. These microbes, just like miniature chemical factories, play a pivotal part in the breakdown of fibres, fats and sugars, creating by-products as a result which can either be helpful (like short-chain fatty acids) or less so (like a precursor chemical which is transformed to TMAO in the liver and increases the risk of heart disease).[17] The right balance of gut microbes can ensure fats are efficiently metabolized, preventing prolonged inflammation.

While the precise influence of these microbes on blood sugar remains a subject of study, the broader question of their role in inflammation has been more definitively answered. Indeed, certain microbes are inherently pro-inflammatory, while others are anti-inflammatory. This has been demonstrated in experiments where transferring microbes from mice with inflammation to sterile 'germ-free' mice led to inflammation in the latter with all other factors being exactly the same.[18,19] This not only proves the direct correlation between microbes and inflammation but suggests that the microbes themselves can be the primary cause of inflammation.

The findings are staggering, especially considering the significant role inflammation plays in our long-term health. The idea that the mere transfer of microbes can impact such a complex system within another organism might have been deemed far-fetched two decades ago, but today it's understood that not only do unhealthy individuals with chronic inflammation typically lack beneficial anti-inflammatory microbes, but they also tend to possess microbes that thrive in inflamed environments. These inflammation-loving microbes may even produce substances that further stimulate inflammation.

The majority (around 70–80 per cent) of our immune cells reside in the gut lining, which is in close proximity to our gut microbiome. This leads to constant interaction between them. As we age, especially beyond our seventies, there's a shift in the balance of our immune responses and our microbiome which can result in inflammation and reduced efficacy of immune response.[20] This makes it imperative for us to actively seek to maintain the fine balance between the two.

The balance between our microbiome and immune system helps the immune system fight off infections and tackle potential cancer threats, and prevents overreactions that could result in autoimmune diseases. The decline in this fine-tuning with age can result in heightened inflammation from triggers such as certain foods, alcohol and even medication that might not have been problematic earlier in life. Additionally, the waste products of our metabolism, known as free radicals, accumulate over time, contributing to further inflammation.

By maintaining a healthy microbiome and immune system, we can potentially slow down ageing and prevent associated health complications.

The problem with inflammation and our approach to tackling it arises when pseudoscience promises simplistic solutions. Single superfood solutions, like consuming a goji berry daily for eternal youth, are misleading. The Dietary Inflammatory Index is an example of a tool that tries to quantify inflammation. It's not easy to use and it demonstrates how complex the anti-inflammatory effects of foods are. This tool aggregates extensive research to identify 45 components with either pro- or anti-inflammatory effects. These are all present in a range of foods and we all have very personal responses to them which change over our life course, so my advice is not to try and use the index in your daily life, but simply to eat an abundance of the diverse plants that contribute the most anti-inflammatory effects, such as in the Mediterranean diet.

In conclusion, while ageing brings about changes in our immune system and microbiome, our diet plays a crucial role in managing chronic inflammation and its associated health impacts. Although there isn't a magic pill or superfood to fix all problems, the adaptability of our microbiome provides a silver lining. Unlike our genes, which remain static, our microbiome can be easily influenced and manipulated by our diets and medications, which offer avenues for optimizing the balance of our gut microbes, potentially reducing inflammation and enhancing overall health as we age.

Five top tips for improving your gut microbiome

1. Aim for a diverse range of plant intake of 30 a week of fruits, vegetables, seeds, nuts, legumes and wholegrains
2. Increase your fibre intake
3. Avoid UPFs
4. Eat fermented foods every day – little and often is best
5. Give your gut microbes a break overnight with a daily eating/fasting schedule and avoid eating after 9 p.m.

Prevention is better than cure

The ages of 50 to 70 are a critical time range for us. This is when the effects of the previous decades make themselves heard, and our future health and mortality risks are established. By the age of 65, 80 per cent of adults suffer with at least one chronic disease.

Heart disease and cancer are the biggest causes of death by a big margin for this age group.[21] To prevent them, we can look at the death by risk factor (below) to understand what things we can change to reduce our chances of an early death. Finding out how to reduce this number and improve the number of healthy years we live is a big undertaking, and lots of scientists and companies are trying to crack that code.

FIGURE 13. Number of deaths by risk factor (2019).

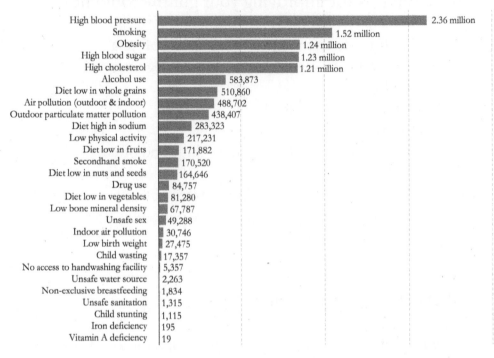

Do supplements work?

Take the VITAL study[22] – a well-designed trial which followed 25,871 men and women over the age of 50 who at the
start of the trial had no heart disease or cancer. They were
given either 2,000 IU of vitamin D3 (higher than the recommended daily dose) or 1 gramme of omega-3 from fish oil.
The aim of the study was to finally have an answer to whether
these two extremely popular dietary supplements reduce the
risk or prevent some of our most feared chronic diseases:
heart disease and cancer.

The findings were underwhelming (but incredibly useful). Taking these supplements daily for more than 5 years didn't really have a benefit, unless you were of African-American origin and male, where vitamin D might improve cancer survival, and omega-3 reduced the risk of heart attacks (but no other heart disease outcome) if you didn't eat any fish. Essentially, it's better to save your money and prevent disease in alternative evidence-based ways.

A recent review of over eighty supplementation studies also came to similar conclusions: supplementation had little to no benefit in preventing a range of health problems like cancer, cardiovascular disease and mortality.[23] More concerningly, this review highlighted that beta-carotene was even associated with an increased risk of lung cancer in those who were high risk.

Reading this book, you might by now be thinking, 'Well, of course taking a supplement of one specific chemical for just five years won't make the difference!' – and you'd be right! By the time we reach the twilight zone, we have rolled the dice many times to get to a certain probability of whether we are likely to develop diseases like cancer. The best known risk factors[24] that lead to death all over the world are:

1. High systolic blood pressure
2. High fasting blood sugar
3. High BMI

These risks alongside smoking all contribute to the biggest global killer: cardiovascular disease. Another thing you might notice is that all, bar smoking, are directly affected by, and can be improved with, good nutrition. This is always one of my most powerful lectures with my medical students as the penny drops when they learn the majority of global deaths are attributable to risk factors associated with diet. Of course, doctors, nurses and other healthcare practitioners should fully understand the importance of nutrition. It's so obvious that delivering timely and practical advice to people could help save their lives.

Here I'm reminded of my beloved papa who died at 63, in full twilight zone territory. He was diagnosed with colorectal cancer at 60 after years of struggling with his weight, yo-yo dieting and trying to find a solution through the type of food he was eating. With no clear guidance, he tried diets which likely accelerated his demise: the Atkins and Dukan Diets, both of which focus on meat and led to initial weight loss and just as rapid weight regain. He didn't have high blood pressure and his fasting blood sugar was surprisingly good for a man who was living with obesity. His cholesterol levels were fine and his fasting triglycerides within normal range. Was he a 'metabolically healthy' person with obesity? No. Basing somebody's health on a handful of clinical parameters is not a holistic way of preventing disease.

His family history and dietary risk were high, he reported being sedentary since his favourite activities – swimming in the sea, skiing and horse riding – were no longer part of his regular life activities since moving to London. And yet none of his healthcare professionals ever intervened to speak to him about his diet, the importance of movement, or to screen him earlier for the cancer that would eventually kill him. In fact, his GP turned him away from screening when he himself asked for it, as he was 'only one year away' from regular screening age. He was told that his blood pressure and blood glucose were fine, if he could try to lose weight that would be ideal, but nothing to worry about. This advice, or rather lack thereof, eventually was catastrophic for him and he is not the only one. We must move to preventing disease, not just treating it after we've ignored all the red flags on the way.

Had he been alive now, I would have organized for him to start his ZOE journey, and no doubt his gut microbiome score would have been very bad. The personalized advice he would have received through the app (he *loved* apps, always ahead of his time) may have made a huge impact on his life course. It has done for my mum, who is my best patient. I wish I knew then what I know now, so that I could have maybe helped to keep him with us for longer, and so my daughters could have met their wonderful Nonno Pietro. So much of what drives me to do what I do now is thanks to him. I hope reading this serves as a lightbulb moment to some of you to take the nutrition of yourselves and your families very seriously. Our lives depend on it.

My tips for approaching conversations around health with a loved one

1. **Talk to them:** ask their thoughts and feelings so they know they are listened to.

2. **Ask how you can help:** there might be something specific they need or want, or a way you can make healthy choices easier for them.
3. **Be understanding:** listen to what they're going through and empathize with their position.
4. **Check their understanding:** make sure they have all the information they need.
5. **Pace the conversation:** give them space when they need it as conversations around health can be stressful and upsetting for some.
6. **Share your feelings:** it's important they know why you're concerned and that you care.
7. **Think before you speak:** take time to consider what you want to say, and how you will say it.
8. **Revisit the conversation:** healthy changes take a long time, and it's a conversation that might need repeating or revisiting.
9. **Try not to blame, criticize or police them:** this can alienate the conversation.
10. **Lead by example:** surround them with positive behaviours to inspire them to make healthy changes.

The view from the top and our 'second spring'

Let's take a step back or forward to your fiftieth birthday. Maybe you celebrate with your best friends, perhaps a party at home with family, a dinner in your favourite restaurant with friends or a trip to a new city with a beloved partner. For many of us, 50 marks the beginning of the second half of our adult lives. Life expectancy in the UK, Canada and Australia is around 82 years of age,[25] with the US lagging behind at 77 years of age, largely due to the opioid crisis. Before you hit 50, you get around thirty years of adult life, then after it you look ahead to another thirty or so. It's the peak of our adult lives, the end of the summer if you like seasons of life as an analogy.

This can be both hugely exciting and quite frightening. What we bring to this point in our lives plays an enormous role in how we continue. Did you sow wisely in spring and harvest plenty in the summer of your life? Are you entering autumn or, better still, your second spring, with plenty of provisions and warm shelter ready for the next adventure? Or if you prefer the mountain climbing analogy, did you make sure to ration your energy and your reserves on the way to the top, knowing that enjoying the summit and making your way back down is just as important and as exciting?

Most of my clients under the age of 30 have a hard time picturing themselves at 55 or beyond. They imagine they would be doing the same thing, perhaps even more things than they're doing now, or they make light-hearted jokes about thinking about it when they get there. It's only when our body starts sending very clear and loud signals that we tend to listen up. A recent example is from a dear family friend who came to me for advice because her hair was falling out in clumps. This had been going on for some months. She asked if I might have some time to spare to help her figure it out. Her GP refused to do blood tests, so she paid to have some private ones and shared those with me. She also shared photos of her hair in the shower, and it was clear that it was distressing to her.

Her blood results were mostly normal; her iron was below optimal which can cause hair loss, but not to the extent she was experiencing. She is in her forties, a healthy weight, and does not have any symptoms of perimenopause – her regular cycles and lack of symptoms also confirming this. Nobody had asked her what she was eating or anything else about her lifestyle. Since her bloods were all normal, she was told she could maybe try expensive PRP treatment, which essentially means injecting her own blood back into her scalp to help heal the struggling hair follicles. Hair loss is by no means a life-threatening condition, but it was affecting her confidence and she had spent a fortune on supplements, private blood tests, and asking different healthcare practitioners for advice.

All it took was a few minutes to find out that she was not eating enough or getting *nearly* enough sleep. She hadn't been advised that food and sleep alone could be the key. She instantly changed her approach to both, making them a priority. Whilst I'm really pleased that she feels better about her hair, I'm even more pleased that she was able to make simple lifestyle changes that have very likely saved her from much more serious health problems in her sixties and beyond. Hair, nails and skin changes are often the first outward visible signs of distress from our bodies, and it pays to listen to them.

It's so important to really evaluate our health status when we enter this window of our lives. The reason I called it the twilight zone is because it's a window when mortality suddenly jumps up. In the UK, we jump from 1.3 deaths per 1,000 men aged 35–9, to 6.6 deaths per 1,000 men aged 55–9.[26] That's a sixfold increase in death at a relatively young age. By the time we hit 74–9 it's 24 deaths for every 1,000 men. In women the rate of death is slightly lower but there is still this obvious upward trend. The UK has introduced regular general health screening for people aged 40+, and many European countries recommend yearly check-ups. I think health screening is one of the simplest ways to identify problems early on, and having a regular set of results to see changes every year is hugely valuable. Intra-individual changes from one time point to the next are what can often uncover an underlying problem much more clearly than a one-off comparison to an average range.

Heart health is the best example we have of how consistent the ageing process is. The vast network of blood vessels in our bodies begins to show signs of ageing as early as our twenties. These vessels, totalling an astonishing 60,000 miles in each individual, begin to stiffen as we age. This stiffening, especially in the minuscule vessels that nourish our organs, poses risks. Blockages can occur due to a variety of factors, ranging from lifestyle choices like smoking to the impacts of a Western diet. High blood pressure, often termed the 'silent killer' because of its frequently undetected presence, is closely related to this vascular stiffening and blockage and is intrinsically linked to diet and lifestyle.[27]

While genetic predisposition plays a role in our vascular health, we aren't entirely bound by our genes. Not only can we halt the damage, but recent insights suggest that we can even reverse some of it. While modern medical interventions like stents or statins are valuable tools in this fight, lifestyle changes are fundamental. Adopting healthier lifestyles, in fact, might overshadow the need for medical interventions in many cases.

High blood pressure is interesting because it doesn't sound

that scary but it clearly has a terrible impact on our body. What do we know about blood pressure regulation and nutrition?

For Curious Bodies

Under pressure

Blood pressure is regulated in two ways. This includes a short-term response known as the baroreceptor reflex, which relies on tiny pressure sensors in our blood vessels. This reflex essentially keeps our blood pressure high enough not to faint when we do things like suddenly get out of bed. Of more critical importance to prevent death is the long-term regulation system known as RAAS. The renin-angiotensin-aldosterone system (RAAS) is a critical player in regulating blood pressure, operating through a complex and methodical cascade of hormonal interactions. Unlike the more immediate baroreceptor reflex, the RAAS system involves a slower, more sustained response.

Renin is a hormone released from specialized structures in the kidney and gets the ball rolling. Triggered by increased salt levels, decreased renal (kidney) blood flow, or sympathetic (fight or flight) nervous system activation, it converts angiotensinogen into angiotensin I. Then, angiotensin-converting enzyme (ACE) transforms angiotensin I into the more potent angiotensin II. These are all hormones that impact our blood vessels. Angiotensin II makes blood vessels narrower and increases the amount of salt that your kidneys hold on to, elevating blood pressure. We now know that just reducing salt consumption does not work in reducing the risk of death associated with hypertension. Unless you add lots and lots to your food, or perhaps drink it because a TikTok influencer has told you to add pink Himalayan salt to your water, you're most likely getting most of your salt from UPFs which always have it added in, even in breakfast cereals or ketchup which are thought of as sweet.

What I find compelling beyond the role of increased salt levels is the role of decreased blood flow and activation of the sympathetic nervous system. The sympathetic nervous system is part of the autonomic nervous system which is essentially responsible for all our involuntary physiological processes: breathing, heart rate, digestion and sexual arousal, for example. The autonomic nervous system is made up of

FIGURE 14. System of blood pressure regulation.

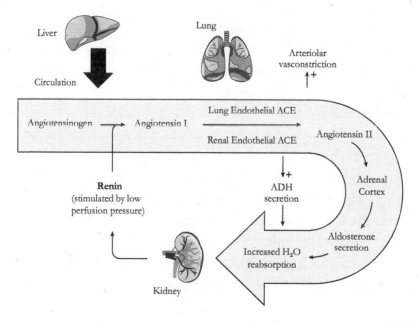

the sympathetic (fight or flight), parasympathetic (rest and digest) and enteric (second brain, gut motility) systems.

Here is my thinking: by the time we reach the age of 50, many of us have spent a good three decades sitting. Sitting at a desk, in a car, on a sofa, on the tube. Many of us have also spent a good proportion of our days stressed. Not the kind of stress that requires the activation of our cardiovascular system (heart and blood vessels) to help us run away from a ferocious predator, but the kind of perceived threat of a missed deadline, annoying partner, bills to pay and high workload. Our body does not know the difference between a perceived threat and a real threat. They are both decoded to real threat signals for our body, activating the sympathetic nervous system to get the hell out of there. Except we don't. We sit, decreasing circulation and blood flow to our bodies, including the kidneys which play a central role for our blood pressure, and activating the sympathetic nervous system to increase a chemical called angiotensin II. Our blood vessels constrict, which means they get narrower, blood pressure rises, and we store the salt we have in our kidneys.

ACE has a dual role: it also degrades bradykinin, a vasodilator (blood vessel relaxer that widens the space for blood to flow) which would normally help our blood vessels relax, so degrading it causes further vessel tightening (vasoconstriction). Angiotensin II also stimulates the release of aldosterone from the adrenal cortex. Aldosterone acts directly on kidney cells, enhancing sodium reabsorption and potassium secretion. This mechanism also links to our pH regulation and hydrogen ion secretion, making aldosterone a key factor in

FIGURE 15. The autonomic nervous system characteristics: 'fight or flight' vs 'rest and digest'.

Autonomic Nervous System
A component of the peripheral nervous system that regulates our involuntary responses including blood pressure, breathing, digestion, heart rate, salivation and sexual arousal.

Sympathetic Nervous System	**Parasympathetic Nervous System**
Fight or flight (for example, a stressful deadline or meeting at work)	Rest and digest (for example, having a bath or meditating)
Muscle breakdown (catabolic)	Muscle building (anabolic)
Associated hormones: Cortisol, Adrenaline (noradrenaline)	Associated hormones: Growth hormone, Dehydroepiandrosterone (DHEA), Melatonin, Testosterone, Oestrogen
Increased heart rate, blood pressure, sweating, blood vessels and pupils dilate	Decreased heart rate, blood pressure, sweating, blood vessels and pupils constrict
Decrease in digestion and sexual function as the body prepares to fight	Stimulates digestion and reproductive system blood flow
Naturally active during the day	Naturally active at night (specifically between 10 p.m. and 2 a.m.)

blood pressure and pH regulation. Potassium is what we lose when we have chronic hypertension, and guess what contains potassium? Fruits, beans, spinach, broccoli, avocado and beets.

Given its significant impact on blood pressure, the RAAS system is often targeted by anti-hypertensive medications aimed at inhibiting aldosterone formation or other components of this system. One of my best, most loyal and adherent clients is my mother. She eats very well, moves every day several times a day and has transformed her life since my father's death, very keen to keep on living. Despite her efforts, her hypertension occasionally comes back, and she's invariably recommended some form of medication. So far, every time it's made a comeback, it's been related to stress and sleep. Every time she reintroduces a daily practice to destress and prioritize sleep, it returns to normal. This is anecdotal evidence, but she is one of three people I work with who see a measurable difference in their blood pressure when they simply choose not to watch the 10 o'clock news and instead read a book or go to bed. Targeting key systems like RAAS through lifestyle changes first, then medication if needed, is a necessary proactive approach to maintaining healthy blood pressure.

The Big C

The other leader of the killer pack is cancer. I've already described how it's affected my family, and it's hard to find a person who hasn't been touched by it. That's because statistically 1 in 2 people will have cancer at some point in their lives, and there are roughly 1,000 new diagnoses made every day just in the UK.[28] The number of cases increases year on year, though treatment success is also improving so that on average a person diagnosed with cancer has a 50 per cent chance of survival.[29] The survival rate varies significantly depending on which type of cancer you have; for instance, cervical cancer has a 10-year survival rate of 51 per cent (i.e. 51 in 100 of those diagnosed live 10 years), compared to pancreatic cancer's rather dismal 5 per cent. The preventability of cancers also has similar patterns, with 99.8 per cent of cervical cancers being preventable compared to only 37 per cent of pancreatic cancer. With bowel cancer, which is what my dad had, 54 per cent of cases are preventable.[30]

If we consider that on average 50 per cent of cancers are preventable,[31] then the 1 in 2 people statistic should be more like 1 in 4. What are the factors driving our risk so high? As we've already touched on, they are lifestyle exposures: smoking, drinking alcohol and our diet are the three biggest contributors to that increase in risk. Whilst smoking won't come as a surprise to anyone, drinking alcohol still might. Drinking alcohol in any amount is one of the biggest risk factors for postmenopausal women and breast cancer. I am lucky to work with women going through the perimenopause and menopause and many of them report to me that they don't tolerate alcohol in the same way they used to at all. This makes a lot of sense in the context of its potential harm. For some, however, alcohol offers a respite and a way to unwind. Unfortunately, that's a more dangerous combination; chronic stress and repeated activation of the sympathetic nervous system are implicated in a variety of effects including hypertension and impaired blood glucose response. If we then have a couple of alcoholic drinks to help temper that, we are adding fuel to the fire.

What booze has got to do with it

I believe that drinking traditionally made wines, with dinner, with friends, has the potential to bring benefits both socially and culturally. The process of growing, harvesting and pressing grapes is steeped in tradition, and celebrating with a small glass of wine can bring a sense of conviviality and joy. I grew up with my big Italian family drinking just one glass of red wine with dinner at a table throughout the meal, and still stick to this tradition now. Unfortunately, society's drinking culture has shifted to more unhealthy patterns, like drinking on an empty stomach after work or a large glass of wine by ourselves at the kitchen counter after a stressful day.

This wouldn't be problematic if it was occasional, say a few times a year, but that isn't the case for many. What I know through my own clients and work I have done with Stride Foundation,[32] a charity which helps addicts looking for support through recovery, which is chronically underfunded in the NHS, is that this type of self-medicating drinking happens *most days* for many of us. This is a product of our environment and upbringing; we are so stressed by our daily environment or feel so self-conscious or simply want to fit in, that we choose to drink as a very effective way to switch that circuit off and remove ourselves from the painful experience of just being. Much as our food environment makes eating UPFs very easy, our drink environment makes cheap, easy-to-access alcohol completely normal. You can buy merchandise that shouts about 'Wine O'Clock', and clever adverts make alcohol appear cool, sociable and fun.

There is a definite shift in younger generations who are side-stepping alcohol for low or no alcohol drinks and finding other tools to deal with their emotional stress. This is an encouraging trend, as is the revival of 'traditional' drinking of some natural wine at dinner as you see in the areas of the world where we see the highest concentration of healthy centenarians, also known as the Blue Zones. This will help in removing some of the increased risk of many cancers, not to mention the societal benefit of reduced drinking. Professor David Nutt is a bit of a legend for being kicked out of government because he ran a huge analysis that showed alcohol to be by far the most dangerous drug we have access to.[33] The headlines read 'Ecstasy is safer than horse riding' and he was booted out for daring to insinuate that drug classifications were not evidence based.[34] Of course he was right, and he has gone on to run some amazing trials that show how some illegal drugs like MDMA and psilocybin (magic mushrooms) can have a hugely beneficial impact on mental health.

In one of his papers[35] he visually plots the risk of harm to self and to society for the most common drugs. The result is an incredibly clear and striking image that highlights how much of a societal problem alcohol truly is. We should be much more careful with alcohol than we have been, and when trying to reduce the risk of cancer, it might be wise to cut it right down since it is, after all, a class I carcinogen and neurotoxin.

FIGURE 16. Different drugs and their harm to users and others.

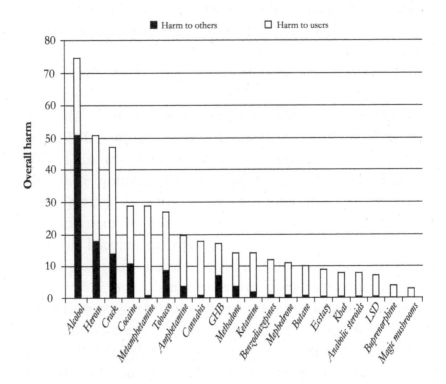

Nutrition and cancer

So what about nutrition and cancer? Consider this in three distinct phases: for prevention, in preparation for and through treatment, and post-treatment recovery. I want to flag here that I am not an oncology (cancer) specialist, so I won't go into detail about the nutritional needs of patients undergoing chemotherapy, radiotherapy or immunotherapy, because it is outside my professional remit. It is also highly personal and dependent on factors such as type of cancer, type of treatment, nutritional status at the onset of treatment and prognosis.

I have clients who have come to me around the time of diagnosis and I support them in getting ready for treatment as part of a multi-disciplinary team at Curia Health.

What I am passionate about is that people should know that there is good evidence to suggest that what we eat is important. Too often, cancer patients are told to 'eat whatever they like'. I think this comes from a good place of avoiding added stress. It's also perhaps not as impactful on likelihood of survival as the other factors, so people don't bring it up to avoid confusion. I think this is changing too, and as more targeted therapies become available, making sure we have good nutritional status can actually make a big difference to how we feel, survive and recover. And even if we don't survive, we can improve our quality of life for the last months.

There is good science on how dietary patterns can help to prevent cancer,[36] and there is an exciting area of research emerging for the preparation of the gut microbiome to maximize the chances of positive immunotherapy outcomes. Processed meats like salami, spam and industrial sausages multiple times a week, are associated with a higher risk of cancer.[37] One bacon sandwich is not going to seal your fate, but daily bacon sarnies have an impact. The rest of the evidence is more around dietary patterns than individual foods themselves.

It's important to remember that dietary patterns and consistency are important and there are no superfoods. Judging by the internet, you'd think there is a specific list of foods to avoid and a specific list of foods to eat every day to help prevent and beat cancer. Of all the confirmed human carcinogens by IARC (the WHO's international agency for research on cancer), of which there are many,[38] smoking, alcohol and eating processed meats are the ones that make the list which are relevant to our lifestyle. Chinese salted fish and betel nut are two others, though I haven't come across them very much in my time so far. The others are mostly viruses (HIV, HPV, Hepatitis B and C, Epstein-Barre Virus amongst others) and lots of environmental exposures that make up what I refer to as the Exposome – the topic of a whole book by itself. On this slightly terrifying graphic, you can also see some green exposures, which are the protective ones. Amongst the protective exposures are things like having a healthy body composition, regular physical exercise, quitting smoking and screening for cancers with things like cervical screening and mammograms.

You'd be forgiven for thinking that food has no role to play in preventing these cancers, but again we go back to the complexities of nutrition epidemiology. There are lots of studies that show how a diet high in fibre, fruits and vegetables, extra virgin olive oil, nuts and seeds is associated with a reduced risk of colon cancer, for example. It's very tricky to pin down foods as causing cancer or directly causing a decrease in risk (which is why the processed meat and alcohol classification is quite impressive!). This is because eating is a complex behaviour and is impacted by so many other factors, including our very individual responses to food. It is easier to find a strong association with the outcome of our diet and lifestyle (i.e. good body composition without excess adiposity/fat tissue) than it is to say exactly which foods are going to decrease risk.

The next time somebody suggests they have the perfect list of foods to eat to prevent cancer, or worse still, they claim to know a special mix of foods or supplements which they conveniently sell to help you beat your specific type of cancer, please beware. Science is moving quickly towards understanding the best approach for improving cancer outcome with immunotherapy, with research pointing to the pivotal role of the gut microbiome in mediating a better response to treatment,[39] and we know that certain dietary patterns like the Mediterranean diet can really help reduce the risk of lots of cancers as well as improve outcomes, but it is not a silver bullet. There is no perfect way of eating, and as we've seen, so many other exposures play a powerful part in causing cancer – diet and exercise are only a part of the picture. One thing is clear, though: reducing our risk of cancer definitely includes not smoking, reducing our alcohol intake, maintaining a healthy body composition, and screening when we are offered it.

Understanding the power of body composition: why muscle matters

Body composition and BMI are not the same thing. There is a lot of debate about BMI – is it useful? Should we care? Why do we still use it? As with lots of other things, the argument around this metric often overlooks what it was designed for. BMI was designed as a cheap, crude measure of body composition to be used to look at population risk of disease and thus public health interventions. It wasn't designed to accurately predict our individual muscle or fat mass, and how can it? The only things it measures are weight and height:

FIGURE 17. Calculation of BMI.

$$BMI = \frac{\text{weight (kg)}}{\text{height}^2 \text{ (m}^2)}$$

Why do we have a tool to measure approximate body composition at a population level? Because measuring *actual* body composition is really tricky at individual level, let alone population level. The technology used to measure body composition is extremely expensive and requires repeated measures as well as skilled technicians to interpret the results. For example, a DEXA scan costs about £150 per body part. To get an accurate idea of your full body composition we're looking at several hundreds of pounds. The less expensive options include skinfold thickness repeated measures and bioelectrical impedance analysis (BIA), which are the fancy electric scales often used in gyms. Skinfold thickness and BIA have an error margin of 5–11 per cent, which is quite a lot when you consider that a 10 per cent difference in body fatness can be the difference between an average person and an athlete. Skinfold thickness measures require meticulous repeated measurements and a lot of skill. I co-led a review of infant body composition and its impact on long-term health[40] and remember thinking how difficult it must have been to get accurate measurements of these babies, kicking and squirming around as researchers tried to measure their body composition.

The problems with BMI can be easily exposed when comparing two people of the same height: a muscular sports-person and someone who doesn't exercise. The increased weight of the muscle in a sportsperson will mean that their BMI will be higher. This isn't just for big, strong rugby players. Usain Bolt, who is incredibly lean, had a BMI of 24.7 when he won his gold medals.[41] This is very close to the 25.0+ which would classify him as overweight, and if a GP saw that on a record without looking at him they might advise him to keep an eye on his weight. In contrast, the person who doesn't exercise might have a lower BMI because they have less muscle, but actually have a far higher proportion of body fat. This means they'll be considerably worse off metabolically and prone to chronic diseases like type 2 diabetes.

The key to understanding the power of body composition is to know two key things: our lean muscle mass is the largest metabolic and endocrine organ in the body. It uses and stores glucose from our bloodstream when we move, and it releases hormones and other proteins to keep our body healthy. The second is that our musculoskeletal mass is what keeps us upright as we age, makes sure we can get up from our chairs and out of bed independently. It keeps us independently mobile.

Now, if we rewind to earlier in this book, you might remember that we reach our maximum capacity of creating muscle mass by the age of 30. From then on, we start slowly losing muscle mass. If we don't work to maintain, challenge and grow our muscles into older age, we will lose this power-ful ally that reduces our risk of cancer and metabolic disease and maintains our independence. At this point, you might be googling me to see whether I am a body builder of some sort. I am not. The muscle mass I am talking about here is not for show, it's functional. It's the kind that helps us move our bodies independently across all planes, the kind that toddlers and young children so naturally use in their everyday movements: climbing, bending, squatting, jumping and lifting. When I talk about keeping our muscles active, I want you to picture a young child playing and climbing, not Arnold Schwarzenegger (no offence to Arnie).

Using your waist circumference as a measure of healthy body composition

For the first time, the National Institute of Clinical Excellence (NICE) has recommended using waist-to-height ratio as a proxy measure for central adiposity[42] – unhealthy fat stored around your organs. Using this measure is useful to assess and predict the risk of type 2 diabetes, high blood pressure and heart disease, and you don't even need a tape measure to do it!

Simply take a piece of string and measure your height standing up straight from feet to top of your head. Cut that string to your height and fold it exactly in half. If you can wrap the halved string around your waist, you have a lower risk of cardio-metabolic disease. If you can't, try to make some simple changes:

- Eat all your food between 9 a.m.–7 p.m. most days

- Move your body every day

- Try to eat your food more slowly, taking your time between mouthfuls

- Think vegetables first: start all your meals with fibre

A healthy waist-to-height ratio is a critically important target for better health, making sure we reach a healthy weight and a healthy waist helps to avoid being over or underweight, both of which are dangerous for health.[43]

Move your body

Prioritizing various forms of daily movement is one of the best ways to improve our trajectory of ageing. My clients who are verging on metabolic disease often like to remind me that they go to the gym once, twice or three times every week. They sometimes have excellent specialist personal trainers. It's no surprise they get annoyed with me when I say, 'That's great, but what are you doing to move every day?' Moving intensely for three hours every week is fantastic for lots of reasons, but it does not constitute an active daily life-style. Our bodies and our metabolism are designed to move throughout the day, even if we have periods of inactivity like resting, working and eating.

A good way to think about daily movement is to split up

our average day into how we spend each hour. Eight hours are for sleeping and another eight are for working. The remaining eight hours are needed to live our life. If I made a guide for my average weekday it would look like this:

FIGURE 18. My average weekday routine.

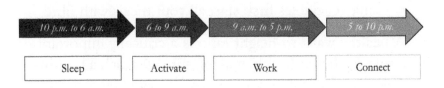

| 10 p.m. to 6 a.m. | 6 to 9 a.m. | 9 a.m. to 5 p.m. | 5 to 10 p.m. |
| Sleep | Activate | Work | Connect |

I had trouble naming the fourth quadrant because so much happens in that time frame. First of all, I rarely finish work by 5 p.m., so there's some work in there. It's also the time when I connect with my children and husband, and perhaps my mum, friends or brother. In that window we are also preparing and sharing food, doing homework, playing hide and seek, walking the dog, doing some housework or watching a movie. But not too close to bedtime because we don't want to impact our sleeping window and it's always nice to leave some space for bath time.

When we split our day up so visually, it's easy to see how movement can be overlooked. The best advice I can give – and what I try to do myself – is to introduce movement before work; whether that's the gym, an exercise class, walking the kids to school, walking to commute to work or taking the dog for a walk. The other thing that can make a massive difference is to walk for just twenty minutes after lunch. This is hard to do, especially with a busy work schedule. I aim to put it into my diary and I stick to it as often as possible. In addition to the physical health benefits, this gives my concentration a huge boost too. Finally, the last part of our day – this often involves a commute back home, another dog walk if you have a dog, or a chance to go to a dance class, a run or maybe an online yoga class.

It sounds like a lot, but we have to take the opportunity to move in every window *except* for the sleep window. It really is not worth reducing our sleep to exercise. Sleeping is so important, and whilst we don't all need eight hours, less than seven is likely not to be enough. It's never too late to pop these movement opportunities into your schedule, and it's so helpful to teach our children to do this from a young age. Some of my healthiest clients tell me that they've always gone for a walk when they need to think or solve a problem. More often than not, I think this behaviour which many of them picked up in childhood has served to make them become healthier adults.

How to add more movement to your day

1. Walk upstairs instead of using escalators or lifts
2. Integrate walking, running or cycling into your commute
3. Walk whilst you talk: go for a walk whilst you are on the phone
4. Avoid using the car or bus for distances under a mile
5. Plan walks with friends or family

6. Find a gym or sport you enjoy
7. Go for a short walk before work, at lunchtime, and/or after dinner
8. Park further away or get off a bus stop early
9. Try dancing, gardening, or moving your body in a way that brings you joy
10. Schedule time into your routine to exercise

One thing to note about movement and exercise is that whilst it's important, it is just one of the pillars. There's this funny hierarchy of daily behaviours that is always worth considering. We can't out-train a poor diet, can't eat well to compensate for poor sleep and can't sleep well if our breathing is impaired. This is why exercise is not a good tool for weight loss, and people with poor sleep often suffer from metabolic disease, even if they have a good diet. Sprinkle all of that with our undeniable need for social connection and the huge impact mental health has on our overall well-being, and you have the basics.

Every Body Should Know This

- Chronic diseases associated with lifestyle factors are our biggest killers.
- The twilight zone is the time of our lives in which the risk factors from previous decades can lead to an early death. It's when death rates start to climb from

lifestyle-associated diseases, so it's avoidable with diet and lifestyle!

- Hypertension is the big red flag for upcoming heart disease and it's something we can improve.
- Cancer is caused by lots of different factors; diet and lifestyle are one component we can change.
- Keeping our bodies active and strong is essential for healthy ageing and requires daily commitment. Daily movement includes taking the stairs, gardening, walking 30 minutes every day, learning to dance and using resistance bands at home.
- Drinking alcohol is cultural for many of us. An occasional glass of wine with dinner whilst socializing might work for some of us, but the overall benefit of reducing alcohol is universal and especially helpful for postmenopausal women.
- The twilight zone is avoidable; being aware of it is the first step.

PART 5

To Longevity, and Beyond!

Living a long life has been a primary interest for humanity for centuries. Paintings of the fountain of youth, tales of people living well into their second century and a fascination with those who become great-great grandparents and hold so much history and wisdom within – all bear witness to our desire for a long life. I have huge respect and admiration for older generations, and I am so thankful to have been able to live with my grandparents growing up. One of the most encouraging facts about people in their seventies and beyond is the reported increase in optimism. Though people under the age of 40 tend to be optimistic, and people in their twenties tend to be happy, the happiest group of people are those in their seventies and eighties according to some surveys.[1] Looking into the evidence a little deeper brings up an important point: many, if not all, of these surveys are cross-sectional. Perhaps this idea of a midlife crisis or U-shaped happiness curve is not an accurate representation of people's happiness trajectories.[2] They are asking individuals at one point in time how happy they are, at one age in their life. This means that their reported happiness is not in the context of their lifetime happiness. I can think of many people who are much happier in their fifties than they were in their early thirties. Some of my friends were really unhappy as teens but thrived in their thirties. My maternal grandfather was the jolliest, happiest man you've ever met in his mid-nineties, despite being partly paralysed by a stroke and having only two of his own teeth left.

Happiness is relative. Using an external measure of happiness is like asking someone else to tell you if you're still hungry; it doesn't make sense. Only I can know if I feel happy or not, and although there are some good tools and general guidelines to help us feel happy, getting there is up to us, and it is largely dependent on our circumstances too. Working with people is very helpful in understanding the importance of context, and with context comes the importance of recognizing the difference between living a long life and living a long and healthy life. Many people live longer today than they used to, but the number of healthy life years hasn't increased so dramatically, which means more people are living longer in poor health. This needs to change.

When I was a teenager I volunteered for a wonderful charity called 'Doctors of the World'. They run a clinic for asylum seekers and people with no fixed address in a church hall in Tower Hamlets, a complex part of London that has a high concentration of people living with significant disadvantage. I used to work in this clinic as part of a triage team, screening people to either receive medical care and social support, or legal support and references. I learned so much volunteering there and will never forget one young man in particular. He had arrived by hiding under a large lorry. He was escaping the war in Iraq, desperate to save his own life and that of his younger brother. He was the exact same age as my little brother; he had large brown eyes that were full of sadness. He had come to see us because he was so depressed, he didn't feel he could carry on living any more. He had lost his family, his home, he spoke hardly any English and as a young man on his own was at the bottom of all the lists for housing, help, anything. He didn't want my help with anything other than helping him feel happy again. Was there anything I could do for him to feel better, he asked, and he looked at me and said, 'I just want to feel happy again.'

In theory, he was lucky. He had escaped the war physically unharmed and made it to London where he was in the queue to start a new life. He was young, fit, healthy and able to find his way around the city, accessing services like the clinic where I met him. In practice, he was desperately sad. The context in which he lived was stacked against him, removed from his social networks and having to find new purpose in a life he didn't choose, in a country that was politically at least partly responsible for him having to leave in the first place. I was able to find some psychological treatment for him nearby with an interpreter, and signpost him to more mental health support networks. I never found out what happened to him, but I spent time with him that day, listening, and I never forgot him, the man who was born the same day as my brother, just in a different context.

Measuring longevity

There are countless other examples of people I've met in the two decades since. So many of their stories are etched in my memory, a huge variety of human conditions and experiences. Some people live a dozen lives by the time they've reached the age of 30, others have clear seasons of change. Most people have a lot more going on under the surface than we can imagine. This is why one of my favourite words in the English language is *sonder* (coined by John Koenig in 2012). It means 'the profound feeling of realizing that everyone, including strangers passing in the street, has a life as complex as one's own, which they are constantly living despite one's personal lack of awareness of it'.

Like the continuous flux of cells in our bodies and stars in the galaxies, we are all complex beings living our own personal trajectory. Life is hard for different reasons, usually outside of our control, and we also make choices that either contribute to or detract from our health and happiness. Some people think we go through a common midlife crisis, then mortality starts jumping up in the twilight zone. There are many who feel they are 'too old' at 54 and find themselves still alive and kicking at 86. The widespread interest in longevity and ageing that we see now has brought with it what feels like a wave of positivity around the potential of ageing well. It's even being rebranded by some as 'lifeing' to remove the negative connotations attached to ageing.

Since a young age, I've ascribed to the philosophy that ageing is a privilege that not everyone enjoys. There is no guarantee that we'll make it to 70, 80 or 90. In fact, it may all end soon with a road traffic accident or a sudden unexpected illness. Living like there's no tomorrow doesn't serve us well either way; a life of excess, sleepless nights, no purpose driving our decisions, and a lack of meaningful connections is not what makes for a life well lived, whether it's a lengthy one or not. Similarly, living under a strict regimen of fear-based assumptions of what might happen if we don't follow very specific rules does not bring joy, and will likely result in a lot of resentment if it doesn't pay off. I have known a few people who were always so careful about reducing risk, living a healthy life and meticulously monitoring what they could, and yet developed cancer or a neurodegenerative condition like MND that ended their life prematurely.

The Big Beige

This is probably why the concept of 'everything in moderation' is so popular. It is mostly used when excusing a behaviour we know isn't optimal, and I think it's flawed (you can't 'moderately' smoke and expect it not to have some negative impact). Plus, it's quite boring! I would rather have lots of time with my family, lots of laughter with my partner and lots of opportunity to grow in my work. If everything is in moderation, then it all starts sounding a bit beige. Instead, I prefer to focus on what things should be in abundance, and those that should be less frequent. I would argue that there are some things best left untried because their potential for harm is so high, but it's not always possible to have the foresight or the context to avoid them. For example, we know that people who have several adverse childhood events (ACEs) are 10 times more likely to suffer with addiction from illicit drug use such as heroin and cocaine. We also know that people born in the 1970s and '80s were much more likely to smoke, drink more alcohol and experiment with illicit drugs than people in their twenties now.

The roots of positive nutrition

The principle of abundance over moderation is what underpins the idea of positive nutrition. I love positive nutrition because it's much more likely to work. Cutting out food is incredibly hard; we know it doesn't work thanks to the myriad studies which show how unsustainable calorie deficit and restrictive diets are in the long term. Being able to maintain a strict, exclusive diet beyond six months to a year is extremely rare. These diets are the vast majority of the ones we see around us, and I consider them negative nutrition. They focus on which foods need to be removed, instruct on cutting out entire food groups or indeed, give up food altogether and have a juice instead!

We have moved so far from our evolutionary adaptation that ensured we didn't die from undernutrition, that we now have an entire diet culture focused on encouraging us towards undernutrition – all in the name of reversing the effects of chronic overnutrition from industrially manufactured foods. It's a bit mad when you think about it this way. My grandparents' generation, born in the early 1900s, saw such a phenomenal change in the food environment, it'll be genuinely sad when their stories are no longer being told. My grandfather spoke fondly about his time as a young boy, eating mostly beans and stale bread soaked overnight then spending his whole day on his bicycle, collecting tins to sell in order to make some money for his mother who was raising him and his several siblings alone. My father-in-law has the most incredible life story, and his approach to nutrition and physical exercise has made him into one of the most able-bodied and cognitively sharp 80-something-year-olds I have ever met.

Their stories and those of many others are heart-breaking in many ways – poverty and hunger in childhood are not romantic in any way, but they grew up in a world where you ate enough food, and that was it. There was no constant nudge to eat something else, have more. It simply wasn't an option, and the food that was available was all whole food that was either fresh, tinned, preserved, jarred or dried. There was no such thing as ready meals, breakfast cereals, snack bars and protein shakes. Some estimates suggest that in countries like the US and the UK, we might have fewer centenarians in the future than we have now, partly because of this huge shift in our food environment. Our children eat snacks, sit for hours and hours on end and then eat more food. Adults do the same and we don't realize that we aren't using our bodies to their potential. Some of us aren't even using our minds to their potential; creativity and play is in competition with content which surrounds us from every angle and device.

The principle of positive nutrition can be applied to all of these areas: eat foods that are good for us in abundance, move our bodies in new ways, use an abundance mindset when planning your day – where can you get *more* movement in? How can you make the most of the time you have with your family? Approach this with abundant energy. What is it that makes your mind and emotional health thrive? Is it music or walking in the woods? Or maybe it's painting or meditation, having a hot bath or reading a new novel. We definitely have an abundance of choice, and the positive impact which technology has had is to make so much learning available for free wherever you are. Abundance does not equal excess; it is much more fulfilling and it truly plays into one of the universal truths: time is the only currency that truly matters. How we spend our time shows what we value.

For instance, if increasing my health span and looking after myself so I can be there for my children is one of my core values, but I don't spend even one hour out of every day investing in the things that will result in improved health, my values do not align with my actions. **Nutrition is a form of investment**. By spending time buying, preparing and eating foods that help to nourish us, we are investing in our health with a very good return on investment. A study based on meta-analyses and the global burden of disease data[3] used modelling to predict how changing our diet can really impact life expectancy, and created a fun tool to use with it.[4] Eating more legumes, whole grains, nuts, fruits and vegetables and less processed and red meat is the simplest way to add up to 13 years to your life. The earlier you make the change, the more years you gain, so if I were to optimize my diet now in my mid-thirties I could gain 6.3 years. I actually stopped eating red and processed meat in my mid-twenties and have legumes and whole grains every day, which hopefully means I've added close to 9 years to my life.

Has my approach to life been worthwhile? We won't know until I'm closer to the twilight zone, and I definitely challenged my body with Vodka Red Bull, late nights and an ill-advised stint of smoking cigarettes 'socially' (reader, it's because my partner at the time smoked) in my early twenties. I am by no means a bastion of optimal health exposures from birth; in fact, I am a product of repeated antibiotic exposure due to recurring tonsillitis as a child, and I have clear memories of snacks being a part of my diet. My mother told me recently that weaning recommendations when I was a child were to focus on foods such as pear, lamb, carrots and pasta to start with and not to challenge young tummies with too many vegetables. My poor gut microbiome had little to thrive off if that's the case!

Invest in your health

Having said that, as soon as I became aware, through my education, of the compound effect which lifestyle and behaviours have on health outcomes, I started to adopt a different approach. I remember seeing a graph which outlined how smokers who quit before the age of 30 could avoid over 97 per cent of the increased risk of death that smoking imparts. For me, understanding that my choices give me agency on risk empowers me to make an informed decision. Informed choices feel good because when you make them, they are made with your best understanding of the current situation. This decreases the chances of regret by a lot! I consider myself a contented and happy person, at least partly because I have very few regrets, if any.

I actively invest my time in the things which I believe are worthwhile and which align with my core values. I believe food is a fundamental investment in my health and my family's health, I spend a lot of time working and thinking about my work, because I truly enjoy understanding, contributing to and communicating the power of nutrition and lifestyle change to improve health. I savour the time I spend with my children, and time with them whilst they're still young (and want to spend time with me!) takes precedence over other social commitments. I choose to walk as much as I can, building that time into my day as a priority and also carving out time to strength-train. As we discussed earlier, sometimes there aren't enough hours in a day to do everything, but consistently investing time over years and decades is what results in a good return of investment. Some weeks are better than others and some years are dreadful because things that are out of our control happen all the time. But consistency and accountability are key, especially when looking after our health.

I hope it's clear now that making a change to your diet and lifestyle can make a huge difference, no matter where you are on your life journey. You can enrich your life and your plate with plenty of delicious plant-based foods, getting more fibre through these foods to help you feel happy and full, and lots of health-optimizing vitamins, minerals and high-quality protein from nuts, seeds, legumes and beans, whole grains and good quality fish and eggs. Making movement part of every day by walking more, gardening, dancing or lifting weights, finding ways to move your body that bring you joy, and investing in time spent with family and friends at the same time is another wonderful way to put more life in your years. Starting tomorrow, add some beans to your plate, some buckwheat or barley, some mushrooms and some nuts (if you're not allergic). Most of us don't make these simple additions to our diet and they are proven to benefit our overall health.

The science on longevity, happiness and centenarians is relatively niche, but much of what we know comes from the Blue Zones research and the famous Harvard happiness study. Both pieces of research are longitudinal, meaning they follow people up for decades, looking for the elements which help build a happy, healthy elder. Both pieces of research have made headlines, sold millions of copies of books and spawned Netflix series and podcasts. The message is clear from them both: good food is essential for a long and healthy life, as are social connections and keeping your body active and strong. At the risk of repeating myself, this isn't rocket science. In lots of ways, what science is resurfacing is actually steeped in common sense and biological plausibility. Sleeping at night is good for us; eating and using that energy to move our bodies is good for us; eating foods that we evolved to eat is good for us; spending time with other people is good for us; feeling like we are part of a bigger whole is good for us.

A paradigm shift in ageing and nutrition

The narrative of ageing is experiencing a dramatic shift. Gone are the days when later years were merely seen as a period of inevitable decline. Making changes in your sixties, seventies and eighties can still have a dramatic impact on your quality of life and healthy years lived. Today, as we witness 65-year-olds boasting health profiles similar to those of 55-year-olds, we're awakened to a new truth: ageing can be a chapter of growth, purpose and vitality. One of my favourite studies looking at how dietary change can make a difference to longevity was led by a wonderful group of scientists[5] and looked specifically at how many years of life we could add if we change to a healthy dietary pattern. The results are

FIGURE 19. How many life years can we gain by adopting healthy dietary patterns?

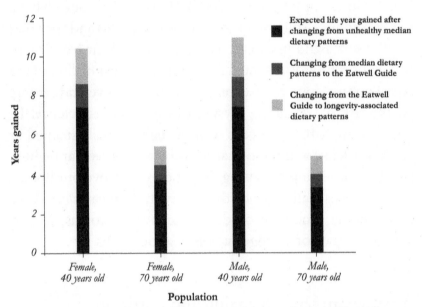

Years gained

12
10
8
6
4
2
0

Female, 40 years old

Female, 70 years old

Male, 40 years old

Male, 70 years old

Population

Expected life year gained after changing from unhealthy median dietary patterns

Changing from median dietary patterns to the Eatwell Guide

Changing from the Eatwell Guide to longevity-associated dietary patterns

Adjusted for socio-demographic area, smoking, alcohol consumption, and alcohol level

amazing! A woman in her forties can gain over ten years of life by switching from an unhealthy standard diet to a healthy, Mediterranean-style diet. A man in his seventies can add five years! It's a wonderful example of how powerful dietary change can be in improving our health at any age.

While modern healthcare, lifestyle choices and societal structures have gifted us increased life expectancy, understanding the significance of diet is critical for increasing our healthy life years. Each meal, snack or drink is a powerful interaction with our body's systems. For instance, while our cells thrive on glucose, overconsumption, especially from highly processed foods, can lead to insulin resistance and metabolic disease. Similarly, our brain is influenced by our dietary habits. Insulin resistance is linked to a steady decline in cognitive function, while eating plenty of omega-3 fatty acids and antioxidants, commonly found in Mediterranean diets, has a protective effect.

This is supported by the findings from the Blue Zones – regions like Greece's Ikaria, Italy's Sardinia, Japan's Okinawa, Costa Rica's Nicoya Peninsula, and Loma Linda, California – pockets of the world where people aren't just living longer, but better.

Central to the longevity witnessed in the Blue Zones are some shared dietary patterns

- **Plant-forward diets**: Beans, grains and an abundance of fruits and vegetables dominate the plates, providing essential nutrients and fibres.
- **Limited meat intake**: Meat isn't the mainstay but rather a side, consumed infrequently and in moderation.
- **Emphasis on healthy fats**: From the antioxidant-rich olive oils of the Mediterranean to the omega-3 laden fish in Okinawa, healthy fats play a central role.
- **Reduced refined sugars**: Natural sugars from fruits are the norm, with minimal reliance on processed sugars.
- **Incorporation of beneficial herbs and spices**: Natural spices, like the anti-inflammatory turmeric in Okinawa, or herbs like the antioxidant-rich

rosemary in Sardinia, frequently make their way into dishes.

- **Eating with intention**: It's not just about what's eaten but how. Mindful eating practices, like the Okinawan 'Hara Hachi Bu', which promotes stopping eating when 80 per cent full, underline meals.

While the Blue Zones are inspiring, longevity's essence goes beyond their boundaries. Diverse nutrient intake is crucial. By expanding our food choices, we ensure a balance of essential vitamins, minerals and phytochemicals. Further, our gut health and microbiome composition, deeply influenced by our diet, has far-reaching implications, from digestion to modulating mental health. A diet emphasizing whole foods while limiting highly processed industrial items can dramatically reduce chronic disease risk, a direct ticket to healthier ageing.

The Mediterranean diet, a staple in many Blue Zones, epitomizes the gold standard in nutrition for longevity. It is underscored by an abundance of vegetables, fruits, whole grains, fish, nuts and olive oil. Besides being absolutely delicious, it's consistently linked with reduced risks of chronic diseases like heart diseases, depression and type 2 diabetes.

The journey of ageing is intrinsically tied to our nutritional choices. To age with grace, vitality and health is not a distant dream but a tangible reality, achievable with well-informed dietary habits. It's not merely about adding years to life, but adding life to those years.

Eating for health at 80 and beyond

The reality is that many of us, by the time we reach our seventies and beyond, have had some form of illness or suffer with a chronic disease. Some have survived cancer, a heart attack or a stroke, others have had total hip replacements, many have struggled with mental health and some are taking medications daily to control symptoms including pain, high blood pressure, high cholesterol levels or high blood glucose. The risk factors earlier in life, if left unchanged, develop into the diseases we've discussed, heart disease still being the biggest killer of them all for men and women. What we eat has a big impact on how we recover from these problems, and I think many people don't realize that our nutrition needs to change a lot in our later life.

Let's start with our gut. As we age, we are more likely to develop diverticula, which are tiny pockets in our gut wall that form with repeated pressure on the gut due to constipation and pressure on the abdomen. More than half of us of us are estimated to have these diverticula by the time we reach 65. The pressure can come from wearing tight clothing, sitting down at a desk with a 90-degree angle or straining when going to the loo due to constipation. Many of us do all of the above for many years, at our desks in offices, and in the way we live our lives. These diverticula don't become symptomatic for the vast majority of us. They just change the elasticity and surface area of our gut wall, much like a balloon that has been inflated and deflated too many times. For a small percentage of people, which increases as we age, the pockets become inflamed and cause severe abdominal pain and diarrhoea as well as bleeding and a rare but potentially life-threatening swelling of the bowel.

Diverticula and diverticular disease are a sign of the wear and tear of our guts, and it's an important reminder that our guts, like every other organ in our body, do age. With this ageing and damage comes a reduction in optimal function. The risk of constipation is greatly increased with age, and it can become life-threatening not to mention extremely unpleasant. Part of the reason why constipation increases with age is the reduced function of our gut, which simply doesn't move as efficiently as it used to, meaning our gut transit time (from fork to loo) is lengthier. Couple this with reduced mobility and a reduced thirst response and you have a perfect storm for constipation. If you are reading this book and you're in your forties, you are significantly more active than you will be in your eighties.

It's not hard to appreciate that if you're not walking up and down stairs, taking a brisk walk to the station or kneeling down to tend to your garden in midlife, you're unlikely to suddenly take it up in your eighties. Gravity and movement is your number one ally in keeping things moving in your gut, whilst sitting down and lying down slows everything. It's also interesting to note how many of my clients and my medical students don't realize that as we age, our bodies become a bit less efficient at reminding us to eat and drink. Our hunger and thirst signals don't have the same impact as they used to, meaning it's not uncommon for older people to forget to drink water for most of the day. In severe cognitive decline and dementia, people lose interest in eating altogether, which can sometimes be the leading cause of their malnutrition, demise and eventual death.

Another important change that takes place in the gut is a

reduced ability to absorb nutrients. In those people who also have dysbiosis, which means an unhappy gut microbiome population, whether due to diverticular disease, IBS or a poor quality diet, there is a reduced ability to synthesize essential vitamins and amino acids, enzymes and hormones. That's a double whammy in reducing available micronutrients and essential functional proteins, and it's why careful nutrition advice can make a world of difference. This often means advising people to eat more food, even if they are worried about their weight. The results can be life-changing: from being tired, demotivated and prone to colds and flus, with the correct nutrition people can achieve vitality, clarity and strength.

I can't stress enough the impact of dehydration here. Easily missed because we just don't feel that thirsty, chronic dehydration can lead to confusion, loss of balance and recurring UTIs. Simple steps to optimize hydration can be life saving in older people, yet it is rarely discussed. Instead, many people talk about hydration in the young, which is much less of a problem due to the robustness of our homeostasis mechanisms when younger. Snack foods and UPFs are often easier to eat: they are ready to eat, they are often easy to open even with reduced hand mobility and they have a softer, consistent texture which is very helpful if you have tooth problems or dentures. Unfortunately, they are also completely lacking in water; in fact, their low water content is partly how they have such a long shelf life. Water makes for an excellent bacterial breeding ground, so industrially made UPFs focus on making the foods dry – biscuits, crispbreads and ready meals alike. Where possible, eating fresh soups, cooked soft legumes, nutrient-packed smoothies, fish and roasted vegetables, stewed fruits and natural yoghurt can make a big difference. Another consideration for the hydration problem is making sure we don't drink too much alcohol, which can cause a decrease in brain size and function, leading to memory loss and falls. Alcohol consumption is something we need to be mindful of throughout life, and especially in later life. It might be a surprise to find out that yearly, nearly 700,000 deaths worldwide are caused by falls, with the majority of these fatal falls happening in people over 60. They are the second leading cause of unintentional injury death after road traffic accidents.

Top five tips for health and nutrition at 80 and beyond

1. **Don't stop moving!**
   Physical activity is vital for physical and mental health, and for reducing the risk of falls, fractures and overall mortality. It's best to stay active to prevent decline. A great way to stay moving at 80 is to do so naturally, by walking where possible.
2. **Remember to hydrate and watch the alcohol**
   Enjoying a drink in the evenings alongside food with friends and family is a great way to stay active and sociable. However, alcohol has more of an impact as we age and can impact our cognitive health and risk of falls. Our thirst response is also less effective, so make sure you're getting plenty of

water, tea and coffee as well as your favourite (small!) tipple.

3. **Find a purpose**
   No matter how big or small, a purpose keeps your mind and body motivated and moving each day.

4. **Prioritize family and friends**
   Community and socializing are hugely important for health and well-being, particularly in older age. Social media and phones can be a great way to stay connected.

5. **Optimize your nutrition**
   Aim to continue the diverse diet I've advised throughout this book, such as increasing plant diversity and reducing UPF consumption. Key changes in older age are that you may naturally reduce the amount you eat since your energy requirements drop as you age.

As older adults, striving to prevent falls seems a good idea. This means staying hydrated and not drinking too much alcohol, keeping well nourished, and being aware of medication that is more likely to make us fall (more on this later). I'm also really interested in how we make movement safer in older age. Too much furniture, too many things that pose a tripping risk and shoes that make it difficult to feel where you're walking are all things we're used to thinking about for our toddlers. But what about in older age? We want to stay healthy and mobile so we should make our homes easy to navigate without the risk of bumps, and walk barefoot, or as close to barefoot as possible, to make sure we get enough sensory feedback from our feet to avoid missteps. A company called Vivobarefoot makes minimal shoes and has shown in a clinical study[6] that minimal shoes improve postural stability when compared to traditional shoes. I only wear minimal shoes and so do my children; I also recommend them to my clients because being able to move safely and without pain is surely one of the biggest prerequisites to keep us moving for longer. I would argue that looking after our feet and moving daily is one of the best ways we can make sure we stay mobile for longer.

Another interesting pivot in older age is that having a higher BMI is actually protective. Closely correlated to ill health in our midlife, having a slightly higher BMI of about 25 above the age of 70 is no longer considered overweight but is actually more closely linked to a longer and healthier life. Suddenly, after suppressing thirst and hunger signals throughout our lives, by ignoring our hunger and satiety signals and drinking gallons of water to reach scientifically unfounded targets often set by companies selling water or water bottles, we are left with a much-reduced sensitivity to these signals. And this is actually quite a big deal. Combining a reduced ability to effectively absorb nutrients with a reduced ability of the gut microbiome to make helpful chemicals and vitamins, and a reduced impulse to eat and drink, all leads to a problem with undernutrition in care homes and in older people who don't have a social network looking after them on a daily basis. When we add the cocktail of pharmaceutical drugs and their effect on nutrient absorption and the microbiome to the mix, appreciation for excellent geriatricians (doctors who specialize in elderly care) starts to soar. And we're going to need a whole lot more of those as our population continues to age!

The importance of resilience

The missing piece in the conversations that take place about longevity and health span, often amongst wealthy, fit and healthy men in their fifties or sixties, is what it's actually like to be elderly. There is a huge dearth of geriatricians, especially when we consider how rapidly we are ageing as a population. Much like paediatrics (the medicine of children), geriatrics comes with very specific tools and tackles unique conditions that aren't found in other phases of life. Many people think of it just as end-of-life care, but it is far more than that. A good geriatrician can literally turn a person's life around, transforming their quality of life and adding years to their life span.

A comprehensive understanding of the biggest risk factors in older age offers some insight into what looking after our health in older age might actually be like. This is not to take away from the inspiring stories of people in their eighties weightlifting in the gym, scaling mountains and living independently, but I'm very conscious that for many people reading this book right now, it might not have happened that way for them, or their loved ones. And the reason I love reading about geriatric medicine, taking additional training courses on the topic, and following some brilliant medics online, is because of the stories of transformation. Transforming our health and well-being is possible at any age, even in the last years of our lives.

There is a delicate balance in later life that has three main contributing factors: ageing-related changes, disease-related changes and medication-related changes. We've touched on some of the ageing-related changes, from loss of muscle mass to decreased efficiency at absorbing nutrients from food and decreased metabolic flexibility. They are all impacted by how we live our lives, the food we eat, what we expose ourselves to, the way we view the world and how we connect with others. Disease-related changes hinge on the physiological effects of having a disease. Hypertension (high blood pressure) changes the way our blood vessels function, and the way our heart and kidneys function as they all try to compensate for the higher blood pressure. This is true for diabetes, other cardiovascular diseases and metabolic disease: all the major diseases of ageing cause changes to our physiology, as well as more 'minor' changes that have a big impact such as loss of hearing. This might seem obvious, and I hope it's making you think back to my rooting principle of homeostasis at the start of the book, but it's sometimes missed as a piece of the puzzle of why resilience decreases with age if we have a disease.

The third piece is the changes caused by medicines. All medicines have side effects. A tablet we take for a headache also has an impact on the whole system. This ranges from the obvious ones like ibuprofen impacts your gut, to the less known ones like antacids and the risk of kidney stones, and the serious ones like paracetamol impacts developing embryos,[7] and statins can cause breakdown of muscle tissues. The problem is that we are all quite used to the idea of taking medication every day for the rest of our lives, especially in later life. As a teenager I took the contraceptive pill every day, and did so for a decade before I decided to stop taking it and find out what my body actually *did* by itself (a very strange and real rite of passage for many women my age).

As an adult I know many people who take antacids, omeprazole, paracetamol, codeine, hormones, antihistamines, antidepressants, anxiolytics, sleeping aids, anti-emetics (for nausea and vomiting) and many other things without thinking twice about it. As we age, taking regular medication becomes more common, and according to the American Society of Consultant Pharmacists, those aged 80 to 84 take an average of 18 prescription medications a year: 18 different medications exerting their own side effects and interacting with each other and with the body in unique ways to exert further effects. It is mind-blowing when you try to think about the pathways that would be involved, if anyone ever tried to map them all together.

So let's go back to the balance, the homeostasis, our body is trying to maintain. Your diet, lifestyle, context, luck and genes have brought you to a certain level of 'changes due to ageing' which your body has managed to keep steady. The diseases and damage you've collected on the way contribute to the 'changes due to disease' which you now have in the balance too. Now let's add in the medications, and the 'changes due to medicines' which are added to every time you take a medicine and it interacts with the other medicines, and with the other changes. There is a tipping point that will be reached at some stage, when the changes all add up together, leaving very little room for error.

This room for error or space for more change is what I like to think of as resilience. Resilience is something we talk about a lot in mental health research, in raising resilient children to become resilient adults. But it's hardly a conversation for the elderly. My favourite analogy for resilience is the bucket analogy. It's not about being tough, or learning to bottle everything up and be strong. It's about building a very sturdy bucket, with a very effective outlet, to process what life throws at us. This analogy works for physical and mental resilience. Let's visualize some examples together.

Let's take the example of two fictional friends in their eighties – let's call them Alex and Bobby. Alex has lived and worked as a farmer all his life, he has an active lifestyle and eats a variety of food from his own land. He has a big family and they spend lots of time together. Money is tight so Alex hasn't always had access to the best medical care, and he suffers with some gum disease and some joint pain. Now in his eighties, Alex still spends lots of time outside with the animals and helping out with some of the farming duties. He has been prescribed some medication for the joint pain and a pill to protect his stomach from the painkillers. Alex's bucket is quite big and sturdy, and he has a good amount of space left in it before overflow is reached, and his outlet is sufficient for his life inflow.

Bobby is Alex's best friend who lives in the closest town in an assisted living community. Bobby worked at the post office and spent much of his life at a desk eating convenience foods and smoking socially. Bobby has a loving partner who lives with him but sadly has vascular dementia. Bobby is very positive and upbeat but does struggle looking after himself and his partner. With good access to healthcare, Bobby has been on statins for high cholesterol, blood pressure medication for

FIGURE 20. Lifestyle and resilience: a comparison of two friends.

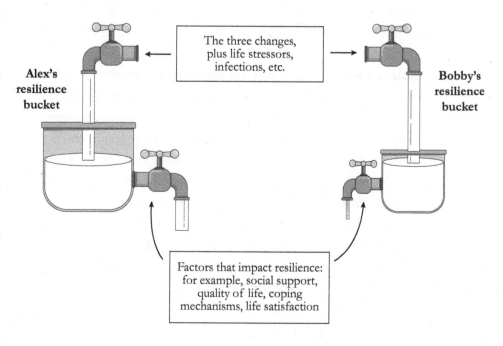

hypertension and insulin for his type 2 diabetes since he was in his early sixties. Bobby also takes antacids and some medication for constipation, having struggled with gut health for a few years. Bobby's bucket is a little smaller than Alex's and it's fuller because he has more changes due to ageing, disease and medicines. Bobby's outflow tap is smaller because he has fewer opportunities to connect socially and his quality of life is affected by his partner's illness.

On the surface, Bobby and Alex are both fairly steady in their health outlook. But what happens when they both catch a cold? A simple viral infection is more likely to tip Bobby's bucket into overflow, resulting in much more severe outcomes than Alex's bucket. And this is where frailty in the elderly comes in. One seemingly 'minor illness' can tumble the balance from independent living and functional ability to being totally dependent on outside help and having an unpredictable recovery. This can be the tipping point of what seems like a sudden change for the worst in older people.

My beloved 96-year-old grandfather went from being a spritely, lively man who loved walking in our garden to look at the flowers, to being completely bed-bound and unconscious in the space of a few weeks. A banal-seeming bout of dehydration (he barely felt thirst and declared the taste of London tap water not even good enough for goats to drink) resulted in confusion, hospitalization, a mini-stroke and eventually his last days spent in a hospice with a view over the gardens where he eventually passed away. In the process, the care he received was terrible and he was written off for end-of-life care far too soon in what ended up being a defining moment for me as I argued with the consultants that they weren't practising patient-centred care. The Liverpool Care Pathway, which is what they had put him on, has now been scrapped. It was the first example I personally lived through of how detached public health systems can become from the people they are caring for, and it is one of the reasons I believe in people having agency over their health and the health of their loved ones.

When all bodily systems are busy keeping a balance on a daily basis, one simple change can have a catastrophic outcome. Knowing what contributes to that tipping point is the first step in preventing it, and understanding that frailty is not a permanent write-off but rather a temporary state that can be

FIGURE 21. Impact of illness on functional ability in older people.

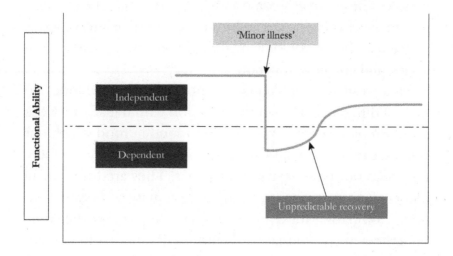

overcome is the second. Dr Elena Mucci is a geriatrician who shares stories of transformation on her Instagram account. She is a brilliant example of a medical professional who has a patient-centred approach, and her account offers an excellent balance of what ageing well can look like, as well as what to think about for a peaceful, personalized and comfortable death.

Microbes, mental health, prunes and polypharmacy

The profound differences in ageing observed among individuals, even among identical twins, underpins much of Professor Claire Steves' research at the Department of Twin Research. Using twins as a backdrop, she investigates the disparities in ageing to shed light on the biomarkers that might underlie these differences.[8] One intriguing find has been the connection between the gut microbiome and diet, particularly the Mediterranean diet. Emerging research even suggests that interventions targeted at the microbiome might yield promising outcomes in ageing and cognitive function.

New research highlights the potential of prebiotics to make a difference in cognitive function within just a 12-week span. Prebiotics are a type of fibre found in food which our bodies can't digest and instead they reach the gut where they feed our beneficial gut microbes. They are found in all plants and encourage the flourishing activity of helpful bacteria. Comparing these findings against a placebo, the study underlines the potential of dietary interventions to combat cognitive decline. This throws into stark relief the significance of intervening early in the ageing process. While interventions at later stages, especially in advanced frailty, seem less effective, starting preventive measures in our fifties or sixties could be game-changing.[9]

Alzheimer's, a major concern for many due to its devastating impact on patients and their families, falls under the umbrella of dementia. Dementia represents a decline in cognitive function to the extent that it impedes daily activities. Alzheimer's, alongside vascular dementia and Lewy body dementia, ranks among the chief causes of dementia. Alzheimer's specifically is characterized by protein deposits in brain cells that, over time, prove neurotoxic. These deposits primarily affect areas responsible for short-term memory.

Crucially, these cognitive changes manifest long after the disease has begun its silent ravage on the brain. By the time symptoms like short-term memory loss become noticeable, the disease might have been progressing undetected for over a decade. Current hypotheses even suggest that these harmful proteins might form in response to gut bacteria, emphasizing the interconnectedness of the gut and the brain.

So, how can we stave off such conditions? Sleep emerges as an important pillar of brain health. Sleep quality and its architecture can aid the brain in clearing out harmful proteins, underscoring the importance of adequate rest. Alongside this, bolstering the immune system through diet and ensuring optimal hearing and vision can make significant contributions to supporting brain function. Recent findings even hint at hearing aids delaying the onset of dementia, emphasizing the importance of sensory inputs in maintaining an active brain.

In essence, the brain, much like a muscle, benefits from stimulation and activity. Just as physical exercise keeps our muscles robust, cognitive challenges and sensory inputs might be the key to a healthier, sharper brain in our golden years. And the role of the gut microbiome in maintaining healthy muscle and a healthy brain is irrefutable, making looking after our gut health an absolute priority. This reminds me of the simple yet amazingly effective intervention of recommending prunes to my older female clients. Not only do they help to regulate bowel movements; they are high in calcium for bone health and very high in polyphenols for additional gut health benefits. A wonderful, affordable food to have in the cupboard and add to our day.

On the opposite end of the spectrum to a few prunes a day to benefit health lies polypharmacy. Polypharmacy is the term used when people are prescribed a cocktail of drugs. The risk of taking drugs that end up causing a fall as a side effect poses a real problem in later life. It's something I was passionate about in 2012, so much so I set up a company and got some seed funding with my idea on how to tackle it. It was too early in my career to pull it off and I wasn't where I needed to be to facilitate the huge amounts of data analysis that I needed. The problem is simple: prescription medications tend to have side effects, especially when they are taken over many months and years. Patients are then often prescribed additional medications to help alleviate the side effect. This changes the picture slightly and with the next visit to the doctor, another ailment is what is being prescribed for. Before long, multiple drugs are prescribed or taken, without a holistic view of how these drugs might be interacting, and how many of the prescriptions are actually addressing side effects instead of solving the health issue at hand.

I think it's important to understand the risk that polypharmacy can pose, but it doesn't mean stopping all your medication. In an ideal world, reducing the need for the drugs would reduce the risk. We've discussed how we can help reduce the need for statins or anti-hypertensives (for high blood pressure) earlier in the book by understanding what our diet and lifestyle choices do to these markers of health. Similarly, we could reduce the need for medication needed to control blood glucose levels if we can prevent or reverse type 2 diabetes. In any case, it's always worth speaking to a doctor or trained pharmacist to review medication and understand the side effects and what to look out for.

The significance of human connection for overall health

Ageing, and its repercussions on our cognitive functions, remains a captivating area of research and one that is hugely important when thinking about health span. Changes in mood and cognition are some of the most prevalent and impactful symptoms of the menopause. Evidence shows that engaging in cognitive tasks not only enhances performance but also brings about structural changes in the brain. While these tasks can be beneficial, the real magic happens with comprehensive activities that engage the entire brain. Physical activity seems to have an overarching influence, potentially due to cardiovascular implications and the hormones produced by muscles during exertion.

The role of social activity cannot be stressed enough. Being socially active is like giving your brain a 'full body workout'. Engaging with your community and interacting with others demand several brain functions, contributing immensely to cognitive well-being. Is it the emotional warmth derived from interactions or the cognitive work of conversing that contributes to a healthier brain? It might be a blend of both. Given our large brains, primarily developed for social interaction, it's conceivable that social activity, in all its facets, is pivotal for mental well-being.

Delving deeper into diet's role, studies emphasize the connection between a diet that is rich in fruits and vegetables and reduced dementia risk. Reducing red meat and switching to a plant-based diet may further delay cognitive ageing. However, research in this realm faces challenges due to the complexities of analysing long-term diet habits and the potential socioeconomic confounders.

Dementia and Alzheimer's have rapidly climbed the ranks and become the second leading cause of death[10] in high-income countries like the UK, the US and Australia. In the UK, it is the number one cause of death for women, above all other causes. I was actually quite shocked to find the WHO graph below which shows how, in just two decades, this terrible disease has increased so rapidly: it has gone from being roughly the eighth cause to the second leading cause. Most

FIGURE 22. Leading causes of death in high-income countries.

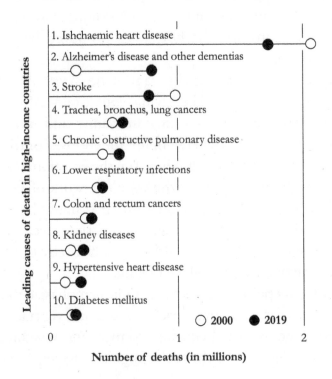

1. Ishchaemic heart disease
2. Alzheimer's disease and other dementias
3. Stroke
4. Trachea, bronchus, lung cancers
5. Chronic obstructive pulmonary disease
6. Lower respiratory infections
7. Colon and rectum cancers
8. Kidney diseases
9. Hypertensive heart disease
10. Diabetes mellitus

Leading causes of death in high-income countries

○ 2000   ● 2019

0   1   2

Number of deaths (in millions)

Alzheimer's and dementia diagnoses are made in people aged 65 or older, with any earlier ones attributed as 'early onset'.

There have been some heart-breaking, beautifully acted films that deal with the topic. From the classic Judi Dench *Iris* to more recent depictions, it is impossible not to feel deeply affected by the progression of these cruel diseases. I remember a lecture when I was an undergraduate student, when our professor chose to show us video footage of one of the most haunting neurodegenerative diseases. It was Huntington's Disease, a rare genetic condition that causes brain cells to die, which usually affects people after the age of 50, when they may have already had children and passed the gene on. The gene is dominant, so all children of sufferers will carry it and go on to develop HD themselves. Disease progression includes loss of motor neurone function similar to Multiple Sclerosis, chorea and ballism, which is a type of involuntary movement that also afflicts those with Parkinson's Disease, and a rapid-onset debilitating dementia that leaves people with HD unable to communicate or recognize their family.

During work experience at a hospital, I spent one day on the dementia ward. At this hospital, like many others, the wards aren't named after the ailment or even the system they are concerned with. Instead, they have names like 'The Red Hyacinth Ward' or 'The Albert Ward', which are not at all helpful when you're 19 and the doctor you're shadowing asks you to observe and suggest what the ward is treating. Some wards are easier than others: the liver ward has people who generally have some level of jaundice, giving their skin and eyes a distinctive yellow or greenish tinge.

The dementia ward was one of those recognizable ones,

but for a different reason. I walked into the ward and couldn't immediately pick out a common trend – people of all ages and physical abilities, no oxygen tubes or tell-tale nil-by-mouth scrawls associated with surgical wards. Then, a man jumped over several beds, ripping past curtain dividers, and grabbed me by the shoulders to tell me to call the police. I very nearly did grab my phone and call the police until I noticed two very calm nurses coming after him. 'I've been kidnapped!' he urged. I looked around and took in the variety of people. One lady lying alone in her bed, completely immobile, turned out to be the first woman to ever receive a PhD from the University of Oxford. Another was a man of 19 who had alcoholic dementia. He had been drinking heavily from the age of 12 and now couldn't remember anything that had happened the day before so resorted to making up different stories to fill the gaps (confabulation) every day we spoke to him. Another still was a woman in her sixties being fed by a kind nurse as she periodically swore at her and looked as though she might punch her.

Dementia and Alzheimer's Disease (AD) are complex, multi-factorial and undeniably cruel diseases that can be heavily influenced by genetics such as in those carrying the APOE e4 gene. The conditions which increase the likelihood of developing these diseases include some familiar names including hypertension, diabetes, obesity, smoking, drinking alcohol, a sedentary lifestyle, social isolation and depression. It's no surprise that some consider these diseases to be metabolic conditions, but there is a critically important point of difference with dementia (60–70 per cent of which is AD), and that is the role of social connection and of sleep. The importance of sleep is huge for good metabolic function and a healthy immune response through a healthy microbiome, and it is even more critical for its role in activating the glymphatic system. This special system switches on during sleep, washing away debris from brain cells, like an efficient sprinkler system that can only function whilst we kip.

Not getting enough sleep, chronically getting less than six hours, is one of the single biggest behavioural risk factors for dementia.[11]

We are facing a problem: the ageing population of today is likely to reach 65 with at least one of the eight main identified risk factors for dementia.[12] Roughly 1 in 3 people don't get seven hours of sleep every night. And then there is the problem of social isolation and depression: there is a mental health and loneliness epidemic at the moment, and we should all be paying much more attention to our own social and emotional health, as well as that of our neighbours and loved ones.

Long live quality relationships

Relationships play an indispensable role in shaping human health, both mentally and physically. The foundation of this sentiment revolves around the quality, not quantity, of relationships. Good, positive relationships nurture our well-being, whereas toxic or strained ones can have negative implications, evoking stress reactions in the body. Stress hormones and the autonomic nervous system are aggravated by negative relationships, which are detrimental to health.

When family relationships become challenging, it's important to manage exposure, perhaps by discussing feelings with other members, and prioritize cohesion and healing where possible. Friends, on the other hand, offer more flexibility. You can distance yourself from friendships that don't contribute positively to well-being, and it's important to teach our children to do so. The evidence is clear though that having a close group of friends that you can rely on and a loving partner to share life with does help improve health and longevity. Having children also improves both, but being in an unhealthy relationship or a household characterized by conflict does not.

The modern age has introduced another layer to relationships: online interactions. A few years ago, the consensus leaned towards online interactions as beneficial. However, the parameters of these studies, often centred around hours spent online, lacked granularity. There is a difference between various types of online engagements. While it's clear that online interactions can be uplifting and engaging, they should not replace face-to-face encounters. Physical interactions have evolved over thousands of years and carry subtle cues and body language that online interactions cannot replicate.

Moreover, online platforms can sometimes become toxic, especially with misleading or harmful messaging. Despite this, the potential positive impact of online connections, when used in moderation, cannot be overlooked. They provide a way to stay in touch, especially in scenarios where physical meetings are not feasible as so many of us learned throughout the pandemic. Still, the healing power of touch can't be overstated, and one of the best pieces of advice for better interactions is to put your phone away on silent where you can't hold it. We have become so used to holding our phones in our hands at all times, it is unnerving to see the impact it has on our ability to truly connect.

Activities that combine creativity with social interactions, such as art classes, dance classes or choirs, are particularly recommended for making good human social connections. Not only do these activities nurture skills and passions, but they also facilitate social interactions. If someone finds themselves isolated, volunteering is a commendable and incredibly effective way to both contribute to society and build connections.

In essence, feeling connected is intrinsic to human health. A sense of purpose emerges as an underlying theme. Retirement, for example, shouldn't be seen as an end but rather a transition to another phase of life with a renewed sense of purpose. Being visible and active, irrespective of age, nurtures mental health.

While the modern age offers the privilege of numerous connections, the emphasis should be on meaningful ones. Such relationships have an undeniable impact on physical health, influencing factors like inflammation in the body. The message is clear: nurturing good relationships is equivalent to nurturing one's health.

One of the most proactive steps anyone can take after reflecting on this is simple: reaching out. Making a call or reconnecting with someone from the past can have a ripple effect. Such actions not only rejuvenate personal relationships but also positively impact the health of both parties involved. The call to action is straightforward – reach out, connect, and cherish relationships for the holistic health benefits they bring.

Every Body Should Know This

- We know more about living a long and healthy life now than we ever have before. Staying physically active, eating a diet rich in plants and nutrient-dense foods, lower alcohol intake and plenty of social connections are key.
- Understanding resilience is critical for improving our chances of surviving unexpected challenges. The more we invest in our health and practices that increase our resilience, the better armed we are for life's challenges.
- Dementia is rapidly rising as a primary cause of death. Decreasing the risk requires a similar approach to the other horsemen of death, heart disease and cancer. Staying connected through volunteering, community service and support networks is proven to improve the quality of later life.
- The food we eat and the company we keep are critical for our health. Choose wisely and spend some time enjoying new recipes with family and friends.
- Medicines save lives but they also have side effects. Be mindful of polypharmacy and aim to come off as many drugs as possible with diet, exercise and resilience practices. Be sure to do this under medical supervision.

PART 6

Health is the New Wealth: This is How You Get Rich

There is one fundamental concept which really helped me to prioritize my focus on health and nutrition. Time is the only real currency we have. You can't buy it, you can't borrow it, you can't foresee how much of it you have left. It is the only truly finite currency which we can choose to invest in what we believe is worthwhile. This is, in my opinion, an essential truth that can help motivate change. At least when it comes to individual agency, we can choose what we spend our time doing and expect a return for it. Consider some obvious examples: spending lots of time on social media seems to result in poorer mental health; spending lots of time playing the piano helps you to become a better pianist; lots of time caring for your health is likely to result in better health. Spending time as a volunteer improves happiness and purpose, and spending time with your family and loved ones increases life satisfaction. Another key idea is that ageing is actually a privilege. Rather than fearing the ageing process and getting 'older', remember that, only four generations ago, it was only the very privileged few who reached their eighties. Life satisfaction and happiness rise as we get older, and our unique perspective on the world, history and the changes we've witnessed become a key attribute that can only come with actually living life for long enough.

It is interesting to note how much money is going into the science of longevity, 'health optimization' and 'life extension'. There is a burgeoning industry of supplements, 'protocols', therapies, technology, off-label pharmaceutical use (for example, metformin supplied to non-diabetics) and a good dose of snake oil. Valued at staggering amounts of money and growing apace, the industry attracts investment both in the personal and business sense. At the moment, it is the arena of white, mostly American, middle-aged men. A lot of them are medics or used-to-be medics. There's lots of money involved and a distinct presence of privilege which, somehow, doesn't make it into the protocols. The truly interesting longevity specialists of our time are arguably those who have thrived into their nineties, despite being relatively underprivileged: the science of resilience and purpose over restrictive diets and expensive supplements.

The new currency

What happens when we look at investing in health at a population level? Public health is the science that aims to address how best to look after population health; it is medicine for the masses instead of the individual. I received my master's in public health in 2010, a year in which the entire structure of the NHS was rejigged. Since then, I feel that public health messaging has been quite clear and consistent for the most part, and public health approaches are pretty predictable. Public health recommendations are evidence based, long-term and often slow to implement. Things that are in the public health domain for decades (for example, we must reduce added sugar in our food) take absolutely yonks to come into policy (for example, the sugar tax) and often on a much smaller scale than recommended by the experts (the sugar tax only covers fizzy drinks and isn't applied to yoghurts, snacks, cereals, etc.).

Between public health recommendations and reality stand many things, including policy (it's hard to persuade politicians to make big moves to improve health if it's not one of their main political interests) and health economics. Health economics, like public health, points to big changes having big impacts but at a much later point. For example, the indoor smoking ban took basically fifty years to come into place when you consider that we knew with certainty that smoking was killing people in 1950 when Doll and Hill published their seminal paper.[1] We have public health and health economics singing mostly from the same hymn sheet: prevent disease years before it develops with changes that can massively reduce risk and are guaranteed to improve outcomes, *but* they need to be made into policies that are actually put into place and actioned. And this is where political will and the short-term nature of our political world clashes with this approach.

If you're prime minister of a country for four years, and want to make some of the changes suggested by public health which will work according to the health economy, you will need to put something in place now for the benefit of the people in 5, 10, 15 or 20 years' time. If that something you put in place is to reduce the sales of UPFs in our supermarkets by incentivizing farming and sales of fruits, pulses and vegetables, it's going to be quite annoying for the companies that make a lot of money selling us UPFs. Those companies that make a lot of money have a lot of money to keep any political party's purse happy, and they might even have a well-paid job for you in four years' time when your premiership ends.

Similarly, if you're a supermarket chain owner who actually wants to make a change to the food environment by reducing buy one get one free deals (BOGOF) or by making unhealthy foods harder to access in the supermarket (middle aisles, bottom shelves where our nuts and seeds and spices often sit), you have to risk that some brands will stop selling their product with you and that some shoppers will get annoyed with you and go to another supermarket to get their BOGOF deals. So what do you do?

Some countries have done a much better job of making public health a priority over and above financial changes. Italy, Spain, France and Greece sell a fraction of the UPFs that we do in the UK and the US. Their political leaders make protecting the food environment a point of difference, with more focus on ensuring equitable access to local foods and supporting agriculture to continue growing and distributing fresh foods to the entire population. The UK is the largest importer of food grown in the EU,[2] more than the entire US, yet it wastes 9.5 million tonnes of food every year.[3] The numbers don't add up, we grow and throw away unimaginable amounts of fresh produce every year whilst 8.4 million people are estimated to live in food poverty. And this isn't about GDP because the UK is technically one of the richest countries in the world, so it is simply a broken system with a lack of focus to prioritize resolving this whole mess.

Rethinking modern food and nutrition

In countries like the UK and Australia, where access to quality food is theoretically good, adherence to dietary guidelines is still surprisingly low. For instance, less than half a per cent of children meet the recommended vegetable intake and less than one per cent of adults meet all the recommended healthy eating guidelines. This trend is not isolated to particular socioeconomic groups; people across the spectrum are falling prey to the allure of the industrialized food system.

The modern industrialized food system, a behemoth comparable to China's GDP, has fundamentally altered our consumption patterns, having profound implications on global health and the environment. This industry, led by large corporations often termed 'Big Food', invests significant resources in designing food products that intentionally stimulate our brain's reward centres, such as the dopamine regions, and encourage us to eat more, even when we aren't feeling hungry. These products offer immediate pleasure, similar to the fleeting satisfaction we get from habits like smoking, drinking or drug use. In the short term, they provide comfort, a satisfying crunch and the right amount of sweetness, but the long-term consequences are detrimental, again drawing a parallel between the immediate satisfaction and subsequent damage caused by other harmful compulsive habits.

These UPFs seemingly bypass our body's natural appetite control systems, making them the go-to option during stressful times. This intentional design and marketing taps into our brain's reward systems, urging us to consume more. Foods that bring us pleasure can be either beneficial, like fresh fruits and vegetables, or harmful, like junk foods. Unfortunately, ultra-processed junk foods are meticulously designed to hit a specific bliss point that is very rarely found in nature, if ever, making them supernaturally delicious. For example, the well-known and much loved hazelnut chocolate ball turns out to be the perfect UPF. It has crunch, it has a smooth, creamy mouthfeel, it has a good solid hazelnut shape to sink your teeth into. It hits the sweet notes but also has depth, delivers high fat, sugar and salt in a tiny perfect package of industrial success with a glossy advertising history. To me, this is a really interesting case study (I also noticed that I suddenly wanted one as I was describing it, despite not having had one for years), but the most striking fact for me was that it is a product that relies on three separate forms of child slave labour: hazelnuts, cocoa and sugar. The problem with UPFs is not only their health impact. Their moral and environmental impact is still hidden. However, understanding the power of dietary choices in preventing or treating illnesses is empowering. When people recognize this, they often make positive changes to their diet – and the realization that it's also helping the planet is a bonus.

The mind–food connection

Depression and anxiety, widespread mental health issues, have historically been studied from a perspective that overlooks the role of diet. During my PhD, I analysed data from an NHS service called 'Increasing Access to Psychological Therapy', launched to help more people access crucial psychological support. One of the biggest takeaways from my research on improving mental health outcomes, and from the colleagues I was lucky to work with on the topic, is how crucial the interplay between poor nutrition and mental health is. Emerging research has shone a light on this relationship and surprised a lot of people. For instance, the SMILES trial gave participants with severe depression a Mediterranean diet intervention and saw promising results, with participants exhibiting a 30 per cent reduction in depression symptoms after just three months.[4] This phenomenal impact is likely mediated by the gut–brain connection, which hinges on the gut microbiota, whose balance can influence our mood. Professor John Cryan is one of the leading experts in the field of microbiota-gut-brain axis, and his research has clearly shown that not only does what we eat and feed our gut microbes directly influence our brain function; these tiny gut bugs can also influence our food choices.[5] Stress-driven cravings are exacerbated by the environment 'Big Food' has created, with products meticulously crafted to maximize our short-term pleasure, often at the cost of our long-term health.

Despite the challenges posed by our food environment, the silver lining lies in our individual agency to make informed choices. Focusing on a plant food first approach, promoting dietary diversity and reducing UPFs, can significantly benefit both our physical and mental well-being. Fermented foods, while not yet directly linked to mental health, can be beneficial for the gut microbiome and our immune system function. And while improving diet can aid mental health, it's essential to strike a balance, ensuring that the quest for a perfect diet doesn't inadvertently lead to disordered eating, especially in conditions like anxiety. The 80:20 rule is one I like to follow myself; I try to eat as well as possible 80 per cent of the time, leaving 20 per cent for the flexibility that life requires.

Imagine for a moment that we could invest in a healthy food environment which maximizes the food we have available to us, feeding everybody in a way that actually improves health and reduces risk. The food we eat is helping us live longer, feel better and be more productive for the economy, running businesses and working more efficiently. Political leaders show a keen interest in this improvement, and we vote for them because we want to live a long, healthy life and not one of prolonged suffering. Nobody wants to go back to the 1870s, where food was all unprocessed but life expectancy was also an average of 37 years – we need to create a new goal. In the 1950s, food scientists set a goal to be able to feed a rapidly growing global population and avoid world hunger. A lesser-known scientist called Howard Moskowitz was tasked with making army food rations palatable so that soldiers didn't suffer the consequences of malnutrition. He is the accidental founding father of UPF: he created the perfect combination and proportions of fat, sugar, salt and satisfying texture variation that helped him achieve his short-term goal, and created a much longer-lasting impact on the food we now eat. We have successfully created lots of hyperpalatable food to (theoretically) make sure nobody goes hungry, and we now have an average of 4,000 calories available to each person living in a high-income country every *day*. Our food environment is too excessive! We overshot the mark.

Now we need to re-evaluate the importance and the impact on health. Being wealthy is no longer just about your bank balance or having a home to call your own. Of course context is still really important, but health is what we can all collectively agree is worth more than anything. Nobody can understand this better than the person who no longer has good health.

Health economics

In the realm of health economics, there exists a fundamental truth: preventing diseases is often more cost-effective than treating them after they manifest. In an era where healthcare costs are skyrocketing and healthcare systems worldwide face immense pressure, understanding the financial implications of disease prevention is paramount.

Disease prevention, which encompasses actions taken to prevent the onset of diseases or halt their progress, stands as a potent weapon against the burgeoning burden of both infectious and non-communicable diseases. From a purely economic standpoint, investing in prevention reduces the future costs associated with disease management, treatment and resultant complications.

*

Let's break down health economics with some tangible examples:

1. **Vaccination:** One of the most cost-effective public health measures, vaccination has eradicated or controlled many infectious diseases that once ravaged populations. By preventing diseases, vaccines save millions in medical costs every year. The costs associated with treating diseases like measles, mumps or polio far surpass the investment required for their vaccines.

2. **Chronic Disease Management:** Non-communicable diseases, such as diabetes, cardiovascular diseases and cancer, contribute heavily to healthcare expenditure. Simple preventive measures, like early screenings, can detect potential issues and mitigate costs. For instance, the cost of regular mammograms is considerably less than treating advanced-stage breast cancer. Similarly, promoting healthier lifestyles reduces the risk of these diseases, slashing future expenses.

3. **Mental Health Initiatives:** The economic implications of mental health issues are vast, encompassing not just treatment costs but lost productivity and earnings. Proactive mental health programmes, offering early intervention and counselling, can reduce these financial burdens significantly.

4. **Antimicrobial Resistance:** Inappropriate and excessive use of antibiotics has led to a surge in

antimicrobial-resistant infections. Investing in antimicrobial stewardship programmes, which guide appropriate antibiotic use, can curtail treatment costs and mortality rates associated with resistant infections.

But the economic benefits of disease prevention extend beyond direct medical savings. Healthy individuals are more productive, miss fewer workdays and can contribute more significantly to the economy. Moreover, households benefit too. Without the looming burden of expensive treatments, families can channel their resources towards education, investments, and improving their overall quality of life.

However, implementing preventive measures isn't without challenges. One major hurdle is the temporal disconnect between investment and tangible results. While costs are immediate, benefits – both health and economic – accrue over time, often spanning years or even decades. This delay can be a deterrent, especially in political spheres where leaders seek quicker returns or in low-resource settings where immediate needs overshadow long-term benefits.

Additionally, while the overarching principle that prevention is cost-effective holds true, it doesn't imply that all preventive measures are economical. It's essential to base investments on evidence-based practices, ensuring that the benefits, both in terms of health outcomes and economic savings, justify the costs.

Where we fail, and what we can do about it

Beyond the physiological scope, the economic ramifications of the chronic disease burden are significant. High treatment costs, decreased workforce productivity and increased mortality threaten global economic stability. Healthcare systems, especially in resource-limited settings, strain under the weight of rising chronic disease prevalence, diverting resources from other critical health issues.

However, all is not bleak. Recognizing diet and nutrition as central pillars in chronic disease management offers avenues for intervention. Comprehensive strategies that promote healthier dietary habits can stem the tide of this burgeoning global crisis. For example, policy initiatives can regulate the content of harmful dietary components in foods, guide agricultural subsidies to favour health-promoting foods, and create consumer awareness through effective labelling.

Furthermore, fiscal policies such as taxing sugar-sweetened beverages can curb consumption and generate revenue for public health initiatives. Public health campaigns can enhance awareness of healthy dietary patterns and the risks associated with poor nutrition.

The global response must be multifaceted, involving collaboration between governments, international agencies, non-governmental organizations and the food industry. Such synergy can guide the creation of environments that promote healthy dietary choices, thereby attenuating the chronic disease risk.

The Power of Your Microbiome

The gut microbiome is a microcosm of its own, an ecosystem within our guts that is as unique to us as our fingerprint. Siblings share more than 99 per cent of their genes but roughly only 20 per cent of their gut microbes. It's fair to say that the role of the gut microbiome has been hugely underestimated until fairly recently. The whole gastrointestinal tract (GI tract) from mouth to anus was generally thought of as a tube that food passes through, with mechanical digestion (chewing) and chemical digestion in the stomach, but the rest was just a tube for getting rid of waste products. Microbes were bad things that caused diarrhoea and other diseases and must be exterminated with the use of antibiotics.

Gut health was not a popular google search term, and colonic irrigation was seen as a perfectly acceptable way to help 'clean out' what we essentially considered our poop tube. Now we know that the gut microbiome has distinct functions that support our health, and washing it out with water is a bit like purposefully flooding a garden: unhelpful and inconvenient. We evolved with our gut microbes to have longer bowels than other primates, so that we can give our gut bacteria time and space to work their magic, breaking down fibres and plant chemicals for us as food moves through the colon. The microbes break down fibres that we completely lack the enzymes to break down, turning an inaccessible source of energy and nutrients into hundreds of different chemicals (called postbiotics or metabolites) for us. The gut microbes thank us for eating these fibre-rich, colourful plants by making chemicals that make us feel and function better. The data is very clear on one thing: regardless of whether we are omnivores or vegan, the more plants we eat, the longer we live, with fewer diseases. No doubt this is at least partly thanks to the role of the gut microbes.

If you want to picture how our gut microbes break down and transform seemingly inert plant fibres, get fermenting. Simply chop some cabbage (I love red cabbage), give it a good rinse and a massage with some coarse salt, then push it down into a clean glass jar. Add some fennel seeds and caraway for added flavour and some shredded carrot if you have one lying at the bottom of your fridge. Add a little water to make sure the cabbage is completely submerged, using a thick external leaf as a natural 'lid'. Pop the jar on the kitchen side or in a cupboard at room temperature and let it ferment. Check on it after a couple of days and you'll see that the colour of the cabbage has changed and there are little bubbles rising to the top of the fermenting liquid, a sign of live fermentation. You might need to 'burp' your jar, letting some air out to avoid too much pressure building up. The bacteria that existed on the surface of the cabbage leaves have started breaking down the fibres and colourful polyphenols in the jar. Thanks to the salt and lack of oxygen, anaerobic fermentation can take place, keeping harmful moulds and bacteria from growing on the cabbage. After a week you will have a jar of fermented food that is completely different in flavour, texture, complexity of nutrients and nutritional benefits. From the humble raw red cabbage, we have a food that delivers added micronutrients, easy-to-digest fibres, probiotic bacterial strains and more metabolites and polyphenols, all thanks to fermentation. Enjoy your ferments daily and store them in the fridge to keep them from fermenting further. Now you know what magic takes place in your gut when you eat a variety of colourful plants!

The Biome Champion – Sauerkraut

Ingredients:
- 1 cabbage (white, red or green – I personally love red)
- 20 g sea salt (or around 2–3 per cent of the cabbage weight)

Instructions:
1. Shred and wash: Begin by shredding the cabbage and then washing it thoroughly.
2. Salt and rest: Place the shredded cabbage in a large bowl. Sprinkle the sea salt over the cabbage and rub it in well. Let the cabbage sit for about an hour to draw out some water.
3. Squeeze out liquid: After the cabbage has rested, use a sieve to squeeze out as much liquid as possible from the cabbage.
4. Add flavours: At this point, you can stir in any additional ingredients you like, such as garlic, onion, chilli, and herbs or spices like dill, caraway seeds or juniper berries.

5. Pack into a jar: Tightly pack the cabbage mixture into a large glass jar or pot. Push the cabbage down firmly.

6. Top up with water: Fill the container to the brim with pre-boiled or filtered water, ensuring the cabbage is fully submerged.

7. Cover: Place a tea towel over the jar and secure it with an elastic band.

8. Ferment: Leave the jar in a cosy place at room temperature for a few days. You should notice signs of fermentation, such as bubbling at the surface.

9. Press and top up: Use a wooden spoon to press the cabbage down daily and top up with water if needed to keep the cabbage covered.

10. Cooler fermentation: After a few days, when the fermentation is active, move the jar to a cooler spot to continue fermenting.

11. Taste test: After about a week, the sauerkraut should be 'al dente' – crunchy and flavourful.

12. Store: Once fully fermented, store the sauerkraut in an airtight container in a cool place for several months.

Summary:
- Shred and wash cabbage.
- Rub in sea salt and let sit to draw out water.
- Squeeze out liquid and add optional flavours.
- Pack into a jar, cover with water, and cover with a tea towel.

- Ferment in a warm place, then move to a cooler spot after a few days.
- Press down daily and keep submerged in water.
- Taste after a week; it should be crunchy and tasty.
- Store in an airtight container in a cool place for long-term use.

And remember, if you're not a fan of the smell of fermenting cabbage, just think of it as the scent of millions of beneficial microbes throwing a party in your future sauerkraut!

The role of the gut microbiome in the gut itself is absolutely fascinating, but the role that these tiny organisms play in orchestrating our health and well-being throughout our bodies is frankly mind-blowing. There is an entire world inside our gut that has its own homeostasis, finding balance every day, its own chemistry and its own ability to change the way we behave to benefit it. Some say we are superorganisms, a home for the trillions of microbes that live in and on us, making us a perfect example of symbiotic existence. Our gut microbes influence our mood, our appetite, our food choices, our immune system, our fertility and even our bone health. Skin conditions like acne and psoriasis are directly linked to our gut microbiome composition, and the likelihood of allergies is mediated by this world inside of our guts.

Microbiome superpowers

The gut microbiome plays a significant role in disease prevention through various mechanisms:

1. **Correlation with Health Markers:** The ZOE PREDICT 1 study[6] found correlations between gut microbes, diet and health markers for diseases like diabetes, heart disease and obesity. By identifying 'good' and 'bad' bugs, the study suggests that manipulating the microbiome through diet can influence these health markers.

2. **Immune System Interaction:** The gut microbiome interacts with the immune system. A healthy microbiome supports the immune system in fighting infections, reducing allergies and defending against ageing and cancer.

3. **Metabolic Regulation:** Microbes interact with and ferment food, controlling the absorption rates of fat and sugar, as well as other nutrients, and affecting metabolism. A diverse microbiome with a good balance of microbes can lead to less harmful effects from the same amount of foods consumed.

4. **Chemical Metabolite Production:** The microbiome produces chemical metabolites like butyrate and vitamins such as K, biotin, folate B6 and B12, which are crucial for immune support

and overall health. Think of it as our own personal pharmacy.

5. **Gut–Lung Axis:** Studies suggest a connection between the gut and lung health, where the immune effects of gut microbiota can potentially reduce the risk and severity of respiratory infections. This became especially interesting during the COVID-19 pandemic, where clear relationships were evident between gut microbiome health and the severity of respiratory symptoms and overall disease outcome.[7]

6. **Inflammation Regulation:** The microbiome influences inflammation levels in the body. A balance of 'good' and 'bad' microbes can reduce chronic inflammation, which is linked to many long-term diseases.

7. **Appetite and Diet Regulation:** Microbes can signal the brain to influence food cravings, appetite and weight gain, promoting the consumption of foods that benefit the microbiome and, by extension, overall health.

8. **Gut Microbe Diversity and Heart Health:** Research has linked gut microbe diversity with heart health, showing that certain fibre-eating microbes can keep blood vessels flexible, which is protective against heart failure and high blood pressure.

9. **Mental Health:** The gut–brain axis, a bidirectional communication system between the gastrointestinal tract and the nervous system,

suggests that our gut health may influence our mental health. Imbalances in the microbiome have been explored in the context of depression, anxiety, and even neurodegenerative diseases.

10. **Longevity:** Thanks to its role in modulating metabolic, mental and immune health, the gut microbiome is a key player in longevity. A long and happy life is intrinsically linked with our body's ability to keep us resilient in the face of disease which is in large part down to a healthy gut.

11. **Reduction of Chronic Inflammation**: Chronic inflammation is a silent threat, associated with ageing and numerous age-related diseases. The gut microbiome can modulate inflammation. A balanced microbiome can potentially reduce inflammation and thereby decrease the risk of diseases, contributing to increased lifespan.

12. **Nutrient Absorption:** The microbiome aids in the breakdown and absorption of nutrients, ensuring that our body gets essential vitamins and minerals. With age, nutrient absorption can decline, but a healthy gut can counteract this trend, ensuring optimal nourishment.

13. **Personalized Nutrition:** As we better understand the interplay between diet, the microbiome and health, there's potential to personalize dietary recommendations based on individual gut profiles,

optimizing health outcomes. ZOE's METHOD randomized controlled trial[6] shows that dietary change can influence gut microbiome composition to include more helpful strains.

14. **Gut-derived Therapeutics:** The gut microbiome could be a source of novel therapeutic agents. Certain bacterial strains or their metabolites might be harnessed for their beneficial properties, be it anti-inflammatory effects, immune modulation or neuroprotective capabilities.

15. **Microbiome Transplants:** Faecal microbiota transplantation (FMT), where a healthy donor's microbiota is introduced into a patient's gut, has already shown promise in treating specific conditions like recurrent *Clostridium difficile* infections. As we gain deeper insights, FMT or refined versions of it might be applicable to a broader range of diseases.

Meet your health mediators

Seminal reviews of the role which our gut microbiome plays point to its role as a mediator of health outcomes. One of the areas I'm especially interested in is how the gut microbiome mediates the beneficial effects of the Mediterranean diet. As you must be aware by now, the Mediterranean diet is uncompromisingly beneficial for all major health outcomes. But why? What is it about the dietary pattern that particularly results in such a positive impact? Studies that have examined the impact which the Mediterranean diet has on the gut microbiome have gone some way in understanding the mediating pathways. In a beautifully designed study looking at how diet can modulate and, crucially, reduce frailty, investigators mapped what effects a Mediterranean diet intervention had on a group of elderly adults. As expected, the diet improved all outcomes, and now we can link these changes in health outcomes to changes in the gut microbiome.

The best part, then, is that we can modify our gut microbiome to help us stay healthy or become healthier at any point in our lives with our food choices. This amazing central control tower that lives inside our guts and that communicates with our entire body through chemical and neuronal signalling can be completely transformed by the food we eat. The ZOE METHOD randomized controlled trial showed just this: giving people personalized nutrition advice based on their own unique biology and microbiome composition resulted in marked improvements in gut microbiome composition and health markers including blood fat and waist circumference, a measure of unhealthy visceral fat stored around our organs. The aim of all this research into gut microbiome modulation, or being able to change our gut bacteria profile for the better, is to prevent disease, improve health outcomes and even reverse certain health conditions. That's a powerful proposition. As I mentioned at the start of the book, changing our genes is difficult, but changing our gut microbiome and what it does for us is actually achievable. What an exciting time we have ahead as numerous trials are underway to understand exactly what makes a healthy gut microbiome and how we can change it to impact a given outcome.

The relevance of the gut microbiome becomes particularly evident when we see its influence on metabolic diseases such as type 2 diabetes and heart disease. For instance, an imbalance in the microbiome, signified by a higher abundance of harmful bacteria, can lead to increased visceral fat and poor blood sugar regulation – both significant risk factors for chronic ailments. Crucially, we've discovered that bacterial diversity on its own is not a good predictor of overall gut microbiome health. For instance, vegans have a lower gut diversity because they have fewer types of foods for gut microbes to feast on. However, their gut microbiome composition is mostly made up of helpful, fibre-loving microbes. This is an example of why looking at diversity alone could lead to misinterpretation of overall gut health; better to have fewer kinds of microbes but most of them helpful in large numbers, rather than having lots of different types, the majority unhelpful. If you were going to set off on a road trip across the Australian outback, you'd be better off with a great crew of helpful people with similar skills rather than a motley crew of people with varying skills but not so great intentions.

Understanding how we measure the population living inside our guts is still not crystal clear. When ZOE updated its gut microbiome database with the latest sequencing technology, 4,992 new microbes were discovered in a sample of just over 35,000 people. That's thousands of microbes associated with our health which had never before been described. We are at a point with gut microbiome science where we know enough to appreciate its critical importance, we're aware of many of the mechanisms by which it is exerting its influence, and we are also still discovering brand-new types of microbes. I imagine it's similar to when people started exploring the Amazonian rainforest: vast, extremely important for the planet, still being explored today many decades later.

The gut–liver axis

An organ that is often overlooked and underappreciated is the liver. The liver could be considered part of the gut along with the pancreas and the gall bladder because they are so interlinked. The food we eat doesn't magically translocate from our gut to our blood; every fat, sugar and protein we consume is broken down by enzymes and taken to the liver for central processing.

As the master metabolic organ, our liver is responsible for the careful balance of sugar levels, making new sugar when we need it and triggering the release of insulin from the pancreas when we have too much. It is also the only organ that can create protein when we need it and package fats and cholesterol ready for distribution throughout the body.

The liver is a magnificent organ that's able to regenerate itself and remove toxins from our blood, and it is in constant conversation with our gut microbiome. It's not hard to imagine how when the gut microbiome is out of whack, it impacts the liver. And when our diet doesn't support liver and microbiome health (they both like a similar diet abundant in plants!), our metabolic health suffers. Non-alcoholic fatty liver disease is rapidly increasing and it is wholly preventable and reversible with diet.

Foods your gut microbes love

Food Type	Examples	Notes
High-polyphenol plants	Strawberries, cherries, red cabbage, black beans, herbs and spices and extra virgin olive oil	Linked to better gut microbial composition, encouraging the presence of more helpful bacteria.
Fermented foods	Yoghurt (with live cultures), sauerkraut, kimchi, kefir, sourdough	Contain helpful probiotic microbes that improve gut microbiome health and immune system modulation.
Prebiotic foods	Fibres	Act as food for the microbiome, stimulating growth of good gut bacteria.
Plant foods	Variety of 30 different plants weekly	Suggested for a rich and diverse gut microbiome.
Whole plant foods	Vegetables, legumes, whole grains, nuts, seeds and mushrooms	Promote a balanced gut microbiome and reduce inflammation.

The insights gleaned from large-scale studies have shown distinct changes in the gut microbiome across different life stages, such as the changes seen in women pre- and post-menopause. Such shifts in the microbiome can have a tangible effect on metabolic health. Additionally, specific bacterial strains have been identified that may predispose individuals to obesity, highlighting the gut's potential role in addressing the global obesity crisis.

With the increasing global burden of chronic diseases, shifting our focus to the gut becomes imperative. The data suggests that optimal dietary practices can substantially reduce the risk of these diseases. One key insight from extensive research is the recommendation to consume a diverse range of at least thirty different plant types weekly. Plants include nuts and seeds, herbs and spices, legumes, beans and whole grains, as well as fruits, vegetables and mushrooms. It's a plethora of delicious foods that change with the seasons. This practice enriches our microbiome and, in turn, offers protection against several chronic conditions.

As the field of gut microbiome research expands, there is also a burgeoning interest in postbiotics. While the health benefits of consuming live probiotics through fermented foods like kefir and kimchi are well-documented, emerging research suggests even inactive (dead) microbial forms can offer significant health advantages.

From birth, the gut microbiome starts educating the immune system. It introduces the immune cells to myriad bacterial components, ensuring that the immune system can distinguish between friendly commensals and potential pathogens. This training is vital as it prevents overreactions to harmless entities, a mechanism underlying allergic reactions and autoimmune diseases.

Beyond its role in education, the gut microbiota strengthens the gut barrier. By doing so, it prevents the translocation of harmful bacteria into the bloodstream. This enhancement involves the production of mucus and support to the integrity of the gut lining, ensuring that potential pathogens are contained within the digestive tract and subsequently expelled from the body.

Furthermore, certain species of gut bacteria can influence immune cell functions in a way that maintains the immune system's balance. For instance, some bacteria promote the development of regulatory T cells, a class of immune cells known for suppressing excessive inflammatory responses. By influencing such processes, the gut microbiome plays a pivotal role in averting conditions like chronic inflammation.

Moreover, a robust and diverse gut microbiome acts as the body's first line of defence by creating a competitive environment. Such an environment makes it challenging for harmful pathogens to establish a stronghold in our system. Through outcompeting these pathogens for nutrients and producing substances that inhibit their growth, the beneficial bacteria of the gut safeguard our health.

Significantly, the gut microbiome's effects extend beyond the intestines. The immune modulation driven by these microorganisms can influence systemic responses. For instance, certain gut bacteria can affect lung immunity, thereby impacting the body's response to respiratory infections.

In conclusion, the gut microbiome is an active participant in our health, playing a cardinal role in shaping and fine-tuning our immune responses. The health of our gut microbiome is intrinsically linked to our overall well-being, resilience against diseases, and our body's ability to mount appropriate immune responses. Therefore, nurturing our gut is tantamount to fortifying our body's defences and lays the foundation for long-term health and vitality.

The Mediterranean diet and the microbiome

As I've mentioned before, the Mediterranean diet is renowned for its health benefits, many of which are attributed to the way it interacts with the microbiome. Here's a summary of the ways each component interacts with our microbes:

- **Plant Diversity and Fibre:** The wide variety of plant-based foods in the Mediterranean diet provides a rich array of fibres and polyphenols. These components are not digested by human enzymes but are instead broken down by gut microbes. This process is known as fermentation. The fermentation of fibres leads to the production of short-chain fatty acids (SCFAs), such as butyrate, which have been shown to have anti-inflammatory effects and are important for gut health. A diet rich in diverse plant fibres can promote the growth of beneficial bacteria and increase microbial diversity, which is associated with better health outcomes.
- **Healthy Fats:** The Mediterranean diet is also high in monounsaturated fats, particularly from olive oil,

and omega-3 fatty acids, found in fish. These fats are not only heart-healthy but also beneficial for the microbiome. They can influence the composition of the microbiome and promote the growth of beneficial bacteria. For example, omega-3 fatty acids have been shown to increase the levels of bacteria that produce SCFAs.

- **Polyphenols:** Polyphenols, which are abundant in fruits, vegetables, nuts, seeds, olive oil, and even red wine, are another key component of the Mediterranean diet that benefits the microbiome. These compounds have antioxidant properties and can modulate the microbiome by inhibiting the growth of pathogenic bacteria and fostering the growth of beneficial ones.

- **Fish and Lean Proteins:** The Mediterranean diet includes regular consumption of fish and seafood, which are sources of lean protein and omega-3 fatty acids. These components can have a positive impact on the microbiome by reducing inflammation and potentially reducing the growth of harmful bacteria.

- **Moderate Dairy and Fermented Foods:** While the Mediterranean diet includes dairy, it is typically consumed in moderation and often in fermented forms such as yoghurt and cheese. Fermented foods contain probiotics, which are live beneficial bacteria that can help maintain a healthy balance of microbes in the gut.

How to nourish your microbiome

Dietary Diversity: One of the primary ways to nurture the gut microbiome is through diet. Consuming a diverse range of foods, particularly plant-based ones like vegetables, fruits, legumes and whole grains, can promote a diverse microbiome, which is often associated with better health.

Probiotics and Prebiotics: Probiotics are beneficial live bacteria that can positively influence the microbiome composition, while prebiotics are food components that promote the growth of beneficial gut bacteria. Foods like yoghurt, sauerkraut and kimchi are rich in probiotics, while garlic, onions and asparagus are excellent sources of prebiotics.

Avoiding Overuse of Antibiotics: While antibiotics are vital for treating bacterial infections, their overuse can disrupt the microbiome by killing beneficial bacteria. It's crucial to use them judiciously and only when prescribed by a healthcare professional.

Limiting Ultra-Processed Foods: Highly processed foods, rich in artificial additives, sugars and unhealthy fats, can negatively impact the microbiome. Reducing their intake and focusing on whole, natural foods can be beneficial.

Physical Activity: Regular physical activity has been shown to positively influence microbiome composition, promoting the abundance of beneficial bacterial species.

Stress Reduction: Chronic stress can negatively impact the gut microbiome. Engaging in relaxation techniques such as meditation and deep breathing exercises, and adequate sleep can mitigate stress's adverse effects.

The gut–brain axis and mental health: an integrated aproach

The gut–brain axis, an evolving concept in the realms of neurobiology and gastroenterology, encapsulates the bidirectional communication between the gut and the brain. With extensive research over the past decades, it has become increasingly clear that our gut and brain, although distinct entities, engage in a profound dialogue that significantly impacts both physiological functions and behavioural processes.

At the heart of this axis lies the enteric nervous system (ENS), often dubbed the 'second brain'. Located within the gut, the ENS comprises a vast network of over 100 million neurons, regulating gut motility, secretion and blood flow. But the ENS doesn't work in isolation; it continuously communicates with the central nervous system (CNS), a link facilitated by the vagus nerve.

The gut–brain communication isn't solely neuronal. Gut bacteria play an influential role. Our gut microbiota, a complex community of trillions of microorganisms, produces various metabolites, neurotransmitters and other bioactive compounds. These substances can influence the brain's function and behaviour by entering the bloodstream or interacting with cells producing hormones and immune system mediators.

Serotonin, a neurotransmitter crucial for mood regulation, provides a compelling example of this interaction. Though widely associated with the brain, over 90 per cent of the body's serotonin is produced in the gut and modulates the availability of the neurotransmitter in the brain through the vagus nerve, highlighting the significance of gut health for emotional well-being and cognitive function.

Central to this discussion is the gut–brain axis and the more complex microbiota–gut–brain axis. The gut and brain communicate extensively, predominantly from the gut to the brain, relaying messages about our dietary intake and any potential threats. Notably, the gut houses a multitude of microbes that primarily break down foods our bodies can't, like plant fibre and polyphenols. As these microbes work, they release molecules that influence various bodily systems, including our immune system, stress responses and neurotransmitter systems. Research suggests that gut microbes can produce neurotransmitters, which can then impact our mood, though most of these don't reach the brain.[9,10] However, they can influence the availability of vital neurotransmitters like serotonin. Interestingly, the majority of the current evidence on the gut–brain relationship comes from animal studies. Still, some human data suggests that disorders like schizophrenia, bipolar disorder and depression may be associated with alterations in gut microbiota.[11] The relationship between diet and mental health disorders like anxiety and depression is nuanced. While there's a clear connection between diet quality and depression, the link with anxiety is less straightforward.[12] Overemphasis on a restrictive diet can lead to orthorexia, an eating disorder characterized by an unhealthy obsession with healthy eating, which can further contribute to mental health problems.

The consensus on dietary advice to bolster mental health revolves around increasing all the foods which promote a healthy and diverse microbiome. As you can probably guess by this point in the book, this includes a diet high in plants, low in UPFs, and with additions of fermented foods. The overarching recommendation is to strike a balance – emphasizing wholesome foods, while also allowing for indulgences, recognizing that no food should be entirely off limits.

Furthermore, the gut–brain axis plays an essential role in stress response.[13] Exposure to stressors can alter gut microbiota composition, leading to a phenomenon called gut dysbiosis. This dysbiosis can amplify stress responses, creating a feedback loop where stress affects the gut and, in turn, the altered gut influences the brain. Such interactions are thought to contribute to various neurological and psychiatric disorders, including anxiety, depression, and possibly neurodegenerative diseases.

In essence, the gut–brain axis serves as a testament to the body's interconnectedness. Understanding this intricate dialogue offers insights into gut and brain health individually, but it also highlights the potential therapeutic interventions that harness the power of this axis. Through modulating the gut microbiome, be it via dietary interventions, probiotics, or other means, there's potential to positively influence brain function and overall well-being.

The gut–brain axis has been a focal point of research for its role in regulating physiology and behaviour. As this axis is unravelled, a significant revelation has been its deep connection to mental health. Building upon the foundational knowledge of the gut–brain interplay, Professor Felice Jacka's work has brought to light the intricate relationship between diet, gut health and mental well-being.[12]

Mind your plate

Dietary patterns play a crucial role in shaping the composition and diversity of the gut microbiota. In essence, what we consume has direct implications for the microbial communities residing within us. These microbes, in turn, produce an array of metabolites and neurotransmitters that can traverse the gut lining, enter the bloodstream, and ultimately influence brain function. Jacka's research underscores that a diet rich in processed foods, sugars and unhealthy fats not only impacts physical health but also poses risks for mental health disorders, including depression and anxiety.

The Western diet, characterized by high sugar, unhealthy fats and low fibre content, has been linked to a reduced diversity of gut microbiota. Such diminished diversity can lead to gut dysbiosis, which has been associated with increased permeability of the gut lining, often termed 'leaky gut'. This condition allows inflammatory compounds to seep into the bloodstream, potentially triggering or exacerbating inflammatory processes in the brain. Chronic brain inflammation is a recognized contributor to several mental health issues.

On the flip side, diets abundant in whole foods, particularly vegetables, fruits, whole grains, lean proteins and healthy fats, support a diverse and robust gut microbiome. Such diets not only foster beneficial bacteria but also provide essential nutrients that act as substrates for the synthesis of neurotransmitters like serotonin and dopamine. Research highlights the profound impact of the Mediterranean diet, rich in vegetables, fruits, nuts, seeds, legumes and olive oil, on promoting both gut health and mental well-being.

Moreover, preliminary studies suggest that improving dietary quality can ameliorate symptoms of depression. Such findings signify that while medications and psychotherapies remain central to treating mental disorders, dietary and lifestyle interventions can offer additional, crucial support.

The gut–brain axis serves as a bi-directional communication channel, and its optimal functioning is contingent upon the nourishment we provide. Embracing a holistic approach to mental health, where diet and gut microbiome are integral components, paves the way for comprehensive well-being strategies. Professor Felice Jacka's work emphasizes that safeguarding our mental health starts, quite literally, from the gut.

Everybody Should Know This

- Industrialization hasn't improved everything. Industrially made food has a place in our future but it needs to be regulated.
- Preventing disease and acting at a public health level makes economic sense.
- The gut microbiome is the most exciting area of nutrition research.
- The Mediterranean diet is the best understood, beneficial pattern of eating we should all be adopting and making available through public health interventions in schools and hospitals.
- The gut–brain axis is part of the answer for the growing challenge of mental health and brain health conditions. Our diet directly impacts our mental health, and our mental health impacts our overall well-being, which is why the gut–brain axis is an important area of research.
- Gut microbes correlate with health markers for major diseases.
- The microbiome supports immune function and metabolic regulation.
- Microbes produce vital chemical metabolites and vitamins.
- Gut health influences lung health and inflammation levels.
- Microbiome diversity is linked to heart health and blood vessel flexibility.

And remember, a healthy gut is like a well-tended garden: neglect it, and you might just find yourself overrun with the weeds of disease rather than the flowers of good health.

Final Word

My goal is to deliver evidence based, practical advice that can serve as a roadmap for anybody looking to improve their health with our best tool: the food we eat every day. There isn't a prescriptive diet, a six-week plan or a specific shopping list, and hopefully now you know why.

Each window of opportunity offers us a clear way to improve our health and the health of our loved ones. Understanding the fundamental role that nutrition plays from the moment we are conceived to the moment we pass away is an exciting and empowering tool. As soon as we appreciate the power of food to make us feel better, perform better, achieve more and genuinely enjoy life more, our relationship with our diet changes. We are all unique individuals with specific needs, personal responses to food and at a discrete point in our lives; one size does not fit all when it comes to health and nutrition. This book helps to map out the main coordinates for good health, the ingredients for a life rich in a variety of foods and nutrients, so that we can all make it work for us, on our own journeys.

I believe that understanding some of the principles of medical science and some of the more interesting physiological marvels that are part of current scientific discovery can help each of us to assess and evaluate advice and act for our own benefit. Knowing what to look out for in a scientific report or how to evaluate other media is another tool that I find helpful so that each individual can make their own choices on which advice to follow. There is so much noise, scare-mongering and opinion dressed as evidence on nutrition and health nowadays, one of the best things to do is to be able to question it independently, and come to our conclusions.

Above all, I hope this book encourages everyone to listen to their own body more. *Every body* does know how to thrive, if we only learn to listen to our body's signals again. We are perfectly created homeostasis masters; we just need to support our biology to do its job. Babies, toddlers and young children are the perfect example of humans who have not lost connection with their body. A toddler will let you know when they're hungry, and they'll also make it clear when they do not want to eat. They nap when they're tired and will express their needs very clearly and often a little too loudly. As adults, we've been told to finish what's on our plate, always eat breakfast, drink water if we feel hungry, eat protein within twenty minutes of going to the gym, start our day with lemon water, avoid nightshades, learn to count calories and make sure to eat little and often (but not to snack!). It's no wonder we've stopped trusting our gut feelings.

Understanding our metabolism, the role of our gut microbiome, the way our hormones interact and how our food environment impacts us is fundamental. An insight into the dietary patterns that we know have an impact on our health and what we can do to reduce our risk of falling ill and cutting our lives short is helpful. Appreciating that life is about consistency and not perfection is essential; striving for perfection kills joy and spontaneity. Nobody wants to get to 110 years old and miserable, and in the same breath, nobody wants to strive for perfection and lose their health sooner than expected, resentful that they hadn't been kinder to themselves along the way. Hopefully the importance of community, the natural environment and our social nature for overall health and happiness is clear. I wish everybody a lifetime of healthy, happy eating for a healthy, happy life.

In the next part of the book, I will go over the main takeaways of each section as an easy-to-use reference.

On reproduction

Reproductive health, encompassing both sperm and egg vitality, is an amalgamation of inherited elements and environmental influences over approximately 90 days of maturation. The endometrial lining's state, crucial for embryo implantation, is influenced by stress, hormones, nutrition and physical activity. Reproductive success is not contingent upon a singular factor, but a combination of several. So, how can we optimize our reproductive potential, especially as many delay parenthood to later life?

At its core, reproduction is the continuation of genetic legacy, with a premium on diverse genetic combinations that yield more resilient offspring. An intriguing dimension to mate selection is our olfactory sense. Pheromones, which often get attention for their romantic allure, play a pivotal role in mate selection. The origins of these pheromones are not clearly established but are believed to be from skin glands, breath, and possibly bodily fluids. Recent theories suggest that our gut and skin microbiome might influence pheromone production. These pheromones' roles are multifaceted, from signalling immune compatibility, a crucial factor in fertility, to relaying genetic and epigenetic information, comparable to a music sheet with unique annotations dictating its rhythm and cadence.

Interestingly, the immune system's relationship with the gut microbiome is symbiotic. The microbiome helps modulate the immune system, and this intimate interaction also influences our scent. One could argue that our body odour is a direct reflection of our internal microbiome's health, akin to sending out a biological status update. This dynamic interplay becomes even more captivating when factoring in the impact of hormones on our microbiome and vice versa, illustrating how interconnected our reproductive, immune and gut systems truly are.

For young adults, this complex interplay is amplified, with hormones, microbes and genetics working in tandem. Naturally, our peak reproductive years are between 20–25. By 30, the chances of conception start declining and by 40, they diminish further. Each menstrual cycle offers a mere 6 or 7 days of optimal fertility, so the odds of conception are akin to winning the lottery.

While the genetic blueprint is essential, we must remember that reproductive success hinges on more than just genetic compatibility. It's a 90-day intense process from germ cell to conception, requiring precise timing and ideal conditions. The in-vitro fertilization (IVF) process has democratized the fertility landscape, but it also underscores the significance of both egg and sperm quality, which can be influenced by lifestyle and diet.

Fertility enhancement often recommends dietary and lifestyle adjustments. Factors such as smoking cessation, moderation in alcohol consumption, and achieving an optimal weight are essential. Nutritional supplements, including folate and iron, can support fertility, with some, like zinc and selenium, having varied clinical backing. Though not often advocated, supplementation can be beneficial during fertility and pregnancy phases.

However, a significant proportion of pregnancies in the UK are unexpected. What happens to those who indulge in occasional excesses without anticipating a pregnancy? The answer is reassuring. Singular missteps are generally inconsequential against the backdrop of an overall healthy lifestyle. It's the consistent, cumulative negative influences that truly impact the holistic symphony of reproduction.

The intricacies of human reproduction are nothing short of miraculous. With just one viable egg and approximately 200 million sperm in an optimal ejaculation, the odds of successful fertilization occurring on the ideal day, paired with a receptive endometrial environment, are astonishingly low. Dr Binazir's calculations emphasized the sheer improbability, suggesting the chance of any individual's existence is virtually zero, taking into account the multitude of factors from our parents' chance meeting to specific genetic combinations.

Male fertility, an aspect often overlooked, plays a pivotal role. Despite societal narratives predominantly focusing on women's biological clocks, male fertility starts diminishing around the age of 35. Particularly in procedures like intrauterine insemination, the man's age emerges as a significant determinant. The Developmental Origins of Health and

Disease (DOHaD) hypothesis posits that foetal programming is a key predictor of an adult's health. An emerging area within DOHaD centres around paternal programming, emphasizing the man's health – factors like diet, stress, BMI, age and exposure to endocrine-disrupting chemicals – as influential in determining sperm quality and overall fertility. Seminal plasma, more than just a vessel for sperm, contains compounds that modify the womb's environment and genetic expression. This underscores that pre-conception health matters for both partners.

This exploration inevitably mirrors my personal perspective, as someone who wanted a family from a young age. It's crucial to understand that fertility, especially with assisted reproductive technologies (ART) like IVF, varies considerably across patients, countries and practices. Some countries frequently employ genetic screening in reproductive processes, while others, like the UK, use it sparingly. The modern narrative, bolstered by celebrities bearing children in their forties, paints a somewhat rosy picture of late-age pregnancies. Companies even promote egg freezing as part of employment benefits. Nevertheless, it's vital to understand the physiological, psychological, emotional and financial implications of fertility treatments and the actual probabilities at different life stages.

On the 'golden window' of opportunity

When a sperm successfully fuses with an egg, an intricate dance of cellular developments begins. Before the embryo implants, the endometrial lining already prepares to nourish it, producing what is described as 'endometrial milk'. This nourishing element signals the womb to make room for transformative growth. Yet the initial stages are fragile. Astonishingly, even during the optimal ovulation period, the chance for a fertile couple to conceive is merely 1 in 5. Furthermore, the first trimester carries with it the shadow of potential miscarriage, with statistics suggesting that up to a quarter of all pregnancies could end during this phase.

Equally significant in this process is the often underappreciated role of the father. Male fertility, especially the quality of sperm, is paramount in conception. Despite society's narrative often emphasizing women's biological clock, it's evident that conception truly is a shared responsibility.

The early weeks of embryonic development rely heavily on the nutrients they inherit from both the sperm and egg. As the embryo transitions into a foetus, the onus of nutrition shifts. By the third trimester, the foetus begins to experience its surroundings more vividly, from changes in light to the flavours of the foods the mother consumes. These flavours, introduced through the amniotic fluid, can even influence a baby's palate post-birth!

The initial weeks can be particularly tough on the mother. With 8 out of 10 women experiencing nausea during the first trimester, maintaining a balanced diet can become a Herculean task. Yet the importance of nutrition cannot be stressed enough. The mother's diet not only supports her own wellbeing but directly influences the development of the baby. Moreover, as pregnancy progresses, the mother's body undergoes profound changes to prepare for birth. For example, the maternal microbiome, or the collection of microorganisms residing in the mother's body, goes through significant shifts leading up to birth. These microorganisms play a crucial role in the baby's initial gut colonization, establishing a foundation for the infant's immune system.

Breastfeeding offers unparalleled benefits for both the mother and baby. For mothers, it aids in post-childbirth recovery, reduces the risk of certain cancers, and even strengthens bones. For babies, breastmilk provides a complex, ever-adaptive mix of essential nutrients, live microbes and immune-boosting proteins. Each feed is unique, adapting to the baby's needs based on factors like time of day and season.

However, the journey to birth and breastfeeding isn't devoid of societal pressures and challenges. From the global market push towards infant formulas to societal expectations, new mothers face a deluge of information and choices. While options like formula milk have their place, it's essential to ensure that mothers are informed about the unique benefits of breastfeeding.

For parents worldwide, introducing their infants to their first bite is a memorable phase, rife with emotions ranging from elation to anxiety. This rite of passage, while undeniably joyous, is often clouded by real fears, such as choking, and the ubiquitous challenges of food messes, waste, and acquiring the seemingly necessary feeding paraphernalia.

Drawing from my extensive experience with numerous mothers and conducting workshops on infant feeding, I've discerned an overwhelming sentiment: the perceived complexity of this pivotal development stage. While I often suggest an uncomplicated approach – a handheld blender or even a fork, a couple of soft-tipped spoons, and some bibs – the one essential investment, in my eyes, is a versatile high chair. Such chairs not only fit seamlessly with family dining tables but also empower the little ones with the autonomy to engage in family meals.

A significant concern in contemporary Western infant feeding habits is the distancing of the child from communal eating. The modern trend of solo feeding, marked by high chairs with individual trays, tends to sever the child's mealtime connection. Undervalued is the significance of leading by example when teaching children to eat. Amusing yet telling, social media videos depict infants eagerly, and often vainly, awaiting food bites from their caregivers. Such moments underline the innate behaviour of children – learning by observing and imitating.

Contrary to segregating children with plastic bibs and solitary meals, immersing them in the collective mealtime experience opens a sensory-rich world. Letting them feel, taste and even playfully squish their food fosters a tactile understanding of their meals. Observing caregivers and peers also helps them discern which foods to embrace and which to approach with caution. However, today's infant feeding trajectory, transitioning from formula feeds to homogenized food pouches, often deprives children of diverse food tastes and textures.

To clarify, I'm not advocating against food pouches entirely – they're convenient for on-the-go snacking. My concern, rooted in clinical observation and data, revolves around the undue reliance on UPFs in children's diets. Disturbingly, UK children derive almost two thirds of their daily energy from such foods, surpassing their counterparts in the US, Australia and beyond. As a proactive step, I encourage parents to reintroduce the joy of natural foods, allowing children to revel in the textures of fresh fruits, the process of peeling an egg, or the unique taste of corn on the cob.

Ensuring safety remains paramount. Differentiating between gagging and choking, understanding food hazards and avoiding risky foods like crisps and olives are all vital. Moreover, maintaining hygiene by thoroughly washing and cooking foods ensures the well-being of the child. While caution is essential, the larger goal should be to enable a rich, exploratory food journey for the child.

Concluding on a crucial note: the introduction of allergens. Past recommendations in the 1990s, advising against allergenic foods, inadvertently escalated allergy incidences. Ground-breaking insights from microbiome science revealed the role of an infant's microbiome in shaping their immune responses. Contemporary wisdom, therefore, endorses early introduction of major allergens, unless the mother herself is allergic. This proactive step can significantly mitigate allergy risks. As parents embark on this gastronomic adventure with their little ones, introducing them to varied flavours, from broccoli to tofu, remember that this is just the delightful beginning – the toddler years await, and they bring a whole new set of challenges and joys.

On childhood and adolescence

The early years of human development are marked by a swift surge in growth, particularly evident in the first two years. During this period, hunger is constant, food becomes the cornerstone of life, and fundamental frameworks of our physical and cognitive being are established. Following this, the trajectory of growth tends to slow down, plateauing especially in the realms of musculoskeletal (muscles and bones) and reproductive organs. It's compelling to note that by the age of 3, a child's brain has achieved 80 per cent of its total growth, establishing its primary structure early in life. While the adolescent years bring about changes in the brain, they are not about growth but more about refinement and fortification of synaptic pathways, known as synaptic pruning. The next significant spike in musculoskeletal and reproductive development emerges around the ages of 12 to 14, commonly recognized as the onset of puberty.

The lymphatic system, though less well-known, plays an indispensable role in our health. This system, comprising lymphoid organs such as the lymph nodes and vessels, is critical in maintaining the integrity of our tissues and is a frontline defender for our adaptive immune system. Contrasting the innate immune system that we are born with and which signals generic alerts like inflammation, the adaptive immune system, developed over time through infections or vaccinations, generates a tailored response against pathogens with greater efficacy.

The evolution of lymphoid organs is a marvel in itself. Prior to birth, specialized cellular clusters initiate the formation of lymphoid tissue within the gut. This connection between the gut and our immune system reinforces the integral part the gut plays in our overall immunity. As a testament to this, secondary lymphoid organs, including structures like tonsils and adenoids, only begin to develop after birth, contributing to the notable growth trajectory observed from infancy to puberty.

Often referred to as the body's 'second brain', the enteric nervous system is a vast collection of nerve cells located in the lining of our gastrointestinal system. It can function independently from the central nervous system and is in a constant dialogue with our immune system. This conversation between the body's immunity and nutrient intake aligns seamlessly with our circadian rhythm, indicating a meticulously orchestrated dance of timing and activation. It not only readies the body to tackle foreign pathogens but also equips it to curb the proliferation of potentially harmful cells from within.

Finally, the role of lymphoid tissue is central to the functioning of our immune system. Its development, which starts early in life, provides the staging ground for immune cells, allowing them to strategize, cleanse the system of rogue cells, and detect internal threats. As children grow, especially during their school years, their exposure to various elements, be it from natural environments or infections, drives the growth of lymphoid tissue. This frequent interaction with a range of pathogens refines and primes the lymphoid tissue, likening it to a series of personalized training grounds, always ready for the next challenge. It's a profound journey of growth and adaptation, from the rapid physical expansions of infancy to the intricate developments of the immune system during the school years.

Growth and development are intertwined with numerous physiological and external factors, with puberty taking centre stage during adolescence. Girls typically begin this transformative phase around the age of 11, while boys embark on it closer to 13. This transition is set in motion by adrenarche, the activation of the adrenal glands. It ignites a flurry of changes, ranging from the emergence of pubic hair and heightened libido to a spike in body odour. The crux of these shifts can be attributed to the adrenal glands producing androgens and various sex hormones. This hormonal fervour attains its zenith by the age of 20 and gradually decelerates thereafter.

Hormones act as the unseen orchestrators of our bodily functions. Integral hormones like the human growth hormone (HGH) originate in the pituitary gland, while insulin is produced by the pancreas. Thyroid hormones emerge from the thyroid glands, with glucocorticoids being a product of the adrenal glands. Prolactin, from the pituitary gland, and gonadal steroid hormones – the sex hormones produced in the ovaries for females and the testes for males – further enhance the symphony of growth. Collectively, these hormones signal tissues throughout the body, guiding them in growth, differentiation and various other functions, culminating in adulthood by age 18.

While hormone therapy has emerged as a remedial measure for certain cases, it's invariably administered under the watchful eyes of paediatric specialists. However, an indispensable element for promoting adequate hormone production is a nutritious diet. The adage, 'You are what you eat,' holds profound relevance, especially during these years of rapid physiological transition.

One of the most crucial phases of this transformation is the 'synaptic pruning' that takes place during adolescence. This phase witnesses a monumental shift in brain structure and function, often occurring in the shadows of academic and societal expectations. Adolescence is paradoxically when society places heavy academic expectations on teenagers, pressing them to store a vast amount of information to excel in examinations. Yet this coincides with the pivotal moment when their brains are pruning away neural pathways deemed redundant. This stage unfolds amidst an onslaught of peer pressure, heightened stress, increased hormonal activity and, often, poor dietary choices.

Unfortunately, teenagers often find themselves overlooked or misunderstood. Like the elderly, they are sometimes perceived as burdens, tricky to handle, and thus left to their own devices. Previously, bored teenagers might have sought thrills outside; however, the digital age now lures them into the realms of social media, online gaming, and the virtual world. This poses concerns, with emerging research suggesting prolonged screen time may push them towards short-term gratification, potentially jeopardizing their judgement regarding exposure to riskier behaviours.

Moreover, the pervasive nature of online advertising exposes them to relentless promotions of fast food, sugary drinks and UPFs. The subconscious influence of these ads cannot be underestimated, as teenagers can unknowingly gravitate towards unhealthy choices due to repeated exposure.

The current food landscape for teenagers is less than ideal, especially during this critical phase of brain development. It's essential that stakeholders, from governments to corporations, acknowledge and address this issue. Initiatives such as Bite Back 2030, founded and run by young people, champion the cause of making nutritious foods accessible for all.

Some nations are already making strides in this direction. Countries like Denmark, Finland, Iceland, Norway and Sweden have instated regulations to monitor junk food advertising targeted at children. France encourages parents to limit their children's intake of UPFs, and Italy boasts a low intake of such foods.

Female adolescence presents its unique set of challenges and considerations. Every month, girls undergo a physiological cycle of creation and shedding of the endometrial lining. This necessitates a consistent influx of essential nutrients. Among these, iron stands out, particularly because iron deficiency and the more severe iron deficiency anaemia are prevalent globally. Heavy menstrual bleeding and its toll on girls' physical and cognitive well-being underline the urgency of addressing this deficiency.

The solution, however, isn't limited to supplements. A balanced diet rich in iron is the most sustainable way forward. In contexts where food scarcity isn't the issue, the emphasis should be on food quality over quantity.

In summary, it's of paramount importance that we return to nourishing our young ones through wholesome foods. Their growth periods are more than just physical expansion; they're transformative intervals that shape their psyche and lay the foundation for their futures. While various factors contribute to overall well-being, food remains a domain within our control. And the current dietary trends among young people warrant a re-evaluation, especially given the profound implications on their mental and physical well-being.

On adulting and midlife

Often, people express astonishment at the heavy emphasis placed on preventing pregnancy during their youth. Traditional educational narratives about sex and fertility predominantly focus on pregnancy avoidance. A more nuanced understanding would involve teaching young individuals about the high fertility chances during their youth and explaining the menstrual cycle's role in fertility. While this information is particularly vital for heterosexual and cisgender individuals, everyone contemplating building a family in the future should possess this knowledge.

The DOHaD theory explores the profound impact of foetal programming on an individual's long-term health. The first 1,000 days of life, often termed the 'Golden Window', are pivotal in shaping the future health trajectories of an individual. As this field evolves, paternal programming emerges as a significant component, offering intriguing insights. A father's health, encompassing factors such as smoking habits, BMI, dietary choices, stress levels, age and exposure to endocrine-disrupting chemicals, has a direct bearing on the health of sperm and seminal plasma. These factors don't just influence fertility but extend their implications to the health of the placenta, potential neurocognitive changes and other disease risks. Semen's role is not merely transporting the sperm; it actively modulates the womb environment and gene expressions, emphasizing the equal importance of paternal health during conception.

Navigating the fertility journey is intricate and deeply

personal, influenced by one's unique experiences and perspectives. Assisted reproductive technologies (ART), like IVF, present their own maze of variability, from patient care, handling of eggs and embryos, cost structures and success rates, to aftercare. It's notable how varied the access and success probabilities are across different countries. Genetic screenings, for instance, are less common in the UK compared to the US. Popular narratives, further propelled by celebrity experiences, may sometimes offer a skewed perception, like the ease of pregnancies in the forties.

The age bracket of 25–35 is often regarded as the zenith of physical capabilities. It's a phase characterized by heightened resilience, strength, fertility and other physical attributes. While happiness metrics might peak later in life, this decade is instrumental in building a robust foundation for later years. The prevailing sentiment is veering towards preventive medicine and the importance of nurturing beneficial habits during this period. Modern trends reveal younger generations refraining more from smoking and alcohol while embracing strength training and fitness routines. Prioritizing holistic health and diversified nutrition is the key to maximizing this period's potential.

Resilience during the prime years can sometimes lead to complacency in self-care. The pitfalls of modern living – excessive alcohol consumption, erratic sleep patterns and unhealthy diets – can have long-term repercussions. Reflecting on personal experiences, it's evident that the vibrant energy of youth can sometimes lead to overlooking the importance of balanced living. However, lifelong fitness and maintaining a sound health profile remain indispensable. A vision for later years should encompass vitality, mobility and independence.

An emerging observation is the narrowing gap between postnatal recovery and the onset of perimenopause. Many women report persistent postnatal symptoms even years after childbirth. The intertwining of these two phases is becoming more pronounced with changing demographics and delayed family planning decisions.

Approaching midlife brings its own set of challenges and opportunities. Career trajectories, family dynamics and self-perception undergo shifts. A comprehensive study indicated that while age-related diseases are on the rise, younger age groups fare better. Nonetheless, lifestyle diseases like dyslipidemia and hypertension show alarming prevalence, underscoring the need for preventive measures. For women, this period also heralds the onset of menopause, with its varied symptoms and challenges. Preparing for this transition is essential, as is looking beyond it, towards a holistic approach to post-menopausal health. The emphasis should be on empowering women with knowledge and resources to navigate these changes.

On the twilight zone

Between the ages of 50 and 70, individuals experience a pivotal moment in their health journey. It's during these decades that the accumulated effects of lifestyle decisions made in earlier years begin to manifest, shaping future health and longevity. Alarmingly, by the age of 65, 80 per cent of adults grapple with at least one chronic disease. Heart disease and cancer stand out as the most common causes of mortality for this age bracket. Many researchers and institutions are delving deep to decipher the best strategies to enhance both the quality and duration of life during these years.

The clinical trials that have taken an analytical dive into the potential benefits of popular dietary supplements including vitamin D3 and omega-3 from fish oil confirmed that dietary pattern is more important than individual nutrients. Engaging 25,871 participants over the age of 50, all of whom were initially free from heart disease or cancer, the VITAL study sought to determine if these supplements could mitigate the risks of these chronic diseases. The results were less than revolutionary. While those who were of African-American descent, male and vitamin D-deficient with a diet low in oily fish (where vitamin D showed potential benefits for cancer survival and omega-3 indicated a reduced risk of heart attacks) showed some positive effect, the study essentially conveyed that these supplements might not be the magic bullet for everyone. It stresses the importance of seeking evidence-based ways to prevent disease rather than relying solely on supplements.

A closer look at global mortality patterns reveals a startling fact: many of the leading risk factors tied to death have a direct correlation with dietary habits. Elevated systolic blood pressure, high fasting blood sugar and increased BMI are noteworthy culprits, all funnelling into the massive threat of cardiovascular disease. Aside from smoking, all these risk factors are intricately tied to nutrition. It's a revelation that has a profound impact on medical education, underlining the paramount significance of nutrition in health. It becomes self-evident that health practitioners need to be well-equipped with nutritional knowledge, as this could be the linchpin in saving countless lives.

On male health

Nutrition plays a pivotal role in men's health, influencing everything from daily energy levels to long-term disease prevention. While our obsession with individual nutrients and supplements has grown, the real key to health lies in the complexity and diversity of our diet. For men, this means focusing on a variety of foods that provide a wide range of nutrients, rather than fixating on specific vitamins or minerals.

A balanced diet rich in fruits, vegetables, whole grains and lean proteins can help maintain muscle mass, support heart health and reduce the risk of chronic diseases like type 2 diabetes and certain cancers which are prevalent in men.

The modern diet, often laden with UPFs, poses a significant threat to men's health, contributing to the rise in obesity and metabolic diseases. It's important to move away from such foods, embracing whole, minimally processed options that are better for both personal health and the environment. Men's nutritional needs change with age, and factors like the microbiome and individual responses to different macronutrients become increasingly important. For instance, some men may handle carbohydrates better than fats, and these personal differences can guide more tailored and effective dietary choices.

Men are more likely to die younger, so the potential of food as preventive medicine is paramount. A diet that is optimal for your unique physiology can prevent or delay up to half of the disease burden from common conditions like heart disease and arthritis. This is particularly relevant for men, who may be at higher risk for certain conditions.

By understanding and utilizing the power of food, men can significantly influence their health outcomes, enhancing longevity and quality of life. The key is to embrace the complexity of nutrition and make informed food choices that support individual health needs and goals.

- Nutrition is crucial for men's health, with a balanced diet supporting muscle mass and heart health, and reducing chronic disease risks.
- A shift away from UPFs to whole, minimally processed foods is essential for combatting obesity and metabolic diseases in men.
- Food serves as preventive medicine, and understanding personal nutritional needs can prevent or delay many common diseases, enhancing men's health and longevity.

On healthy ageing

Ageing is an inescapable natural progression that everyone experiences, yet the effects it has on individuals can differ widely. The differences are shaped by many elements, including our genetic makeup, environmental influences and the lifestyle choices we make. As we delve deeper into the intricacies of ageing, several elements emerge as influential contributors to our quality of life as the years go by.

One of the most significant factors that stands out is physical activity. Contrary to popular belief that primarily mental
activities sharpen our cognitive functions, engaging in regular
physical endeavours, even something as simple as walking,
can have profound benefits on cognitive health. By keeping
track of our physical activity and striving to enhance our daily
movements, we can ensure better health outcomes as we age.

Diet is another critical aspect that holds power over our
cognitive functions. Embracing a diet abundant in fruits,
vegetables and plant-based proteins can offer improved cognitive prowess and decrease the risks associated with
dementia. Making a conscious shift away from diets heavy in
red meat and processed foods to more plant-centric meals
can pave the way for improved cognitive health.

Sensory health also plays a pivotal role in how we experience the world as we age. By ensuring our sensory systems,
specifically our sight and hearing, function at their optimum,
we can interact more fully with the world around us. This not
only fosters better social interaction but also keeps our brains
in peak condition.

The value of quality sleep cannot be overstated when discussing ageing. Sleep is fundamental to our overall well-being.
Investing in rejuvenating, quality sleep has far-reaching
effects on ageing and significantly influences our cognitive
function.

Work and stress are interrelated, and their relationship with
ageing is nuanced. If work instils a sense of purpose and joy
without being a primary stress inducer, it can prove beneficial
for cognitive health. However, chronic stress, whether stem-
ming from work or other sources, can have detrimental health

impacts. Moreover, it's essential to consider the cascading effects of stress, as it often drives individuals towards unhealthy habits, including a poor diet, excessive alcohol consumption and smoking.

Human interaction and sensory input are interwoven into our very fabric. While emotional bonding and warmth from social interactions are invaluable, the cognitive effort required in conversing, understanding and establishing connections makes every social interaction a mental exercise. Hence, maintaining sensory health becomes paramount to optimize the quality of these interactions.

Lastly, one prevailing myth about ageing needs debunking: that ageing is solely about inevitable wear and tear. In reality, environmental factors exert a more profound influence on how and at what pace we age compared to genetics alone. By observing and learning from individuals who age gracefully, everyone can adopt practices to improve their own ageing journey.

In essence, while ageing is a constant process, the manner in which we age is significantly influenced by the choices we make throughout life. Emphasizing physical activity, adopting a balanced diet, maintaining sensory health, prioritizing sleep, managing stress effectively and valuing social interactions can guide us through the challenges of ageing with elegance and vitality.

On building your plate

Every meal offers an opportunity to nourish our bodies using the principles in this book. Building our meals with an abundance of plants, including the trifecta of legumes, whole grains and nuts and seeds, sets us up for delicious, nutritious meals. It's about putting plants first and then adding the rest, whether at home or in a restaurant.

There is always space for some meat, dairy, fish or eggs if you like to eat these foods, as well as refined cabohydrates like pasta, rice or bread, but they are not the majority of the plate and they are not necessary at every meal. This one is up to you and what your body needs!

One plate dishes like risotto, lasagne and fish pies are wonderful and can still be created with these same principles.

FIGURE 23. How to build your plate with a positive nutrition Mediterranean diet approach.

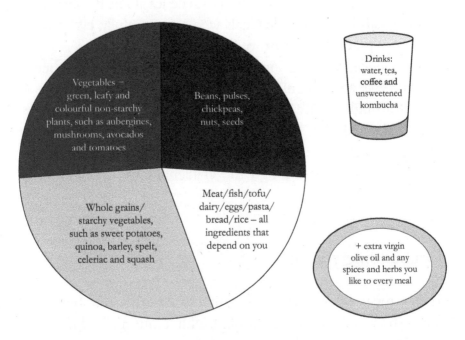

Vegetables – green, leafy and colourful non-starchy plants, such as aubergines, mushrooms, avocados and tomatoes

Beans, pulses, chickpeas, nuts, seeds

Whole grains/ starchy vegetables, such as sweet potatoes, quinoa, barley, spelt, celeriac and squash

Meat/fish/tofu/ dairy/eggs/pasta/ bread/rice – all ingredients that depend on you

Drinks: water, tea, coffee and unsweetened kombucha

+ extra virgin olive oil and any spices and herbs you like to every meal

References

Preface

1. Parnham, J. C., Chang, K., Rauber, F. et al, The Ultra-processed food content of school meals and packed lunches in the United Kingdom, *Nutrients*, 20 Jul. 2022, 14 (14), 296

Introduction

1. Soliman, G. A., Dietary cholesterol and the lack of evidence in cardiovascular disease, *Nutrients*, 16 June 2018, 10 (6), 780
2. Martinez-Lacoba, R., Pardo-Garcia, I., Amo-Saus, E. et al, Mediterranean diet and health outcomes: A systematic meta-review, *European Journal of Public Health*, Oct. 2018, 28 (5), 955–61

Part 1. The Golden Window of Opportunity:
The First 1,000 Days and Early Years

1. Human Fertilisation and Embryology Authority, Fertility treatment in 2012: trends and figures. Available at: http:// ifqtesting.blob.core.windows.net/umbraco-website/1143/ fertilitytreatment2012trendsfigures.pdf [Accessed 14 Dec. 2023]

EVERY BODY SHOULD KNOW THIS

2. Reed, K. E., Carmago, J., Hamilton-Reeves, J. et al, Neither soy nor isoflavone intake affects male reproductive hormones: An expanded and updated meta-analysis of clinical studies, *Reproductive Toxicology*, 2021, 100, 60–70

3. Hempstock, J., Cindrova-Davies, T., Jauniaux, E. et al, Endometrial glands as a source of nutrients, growth factors and cytoklines during the first trimester of human pregnancy: A morphological and immunohistochemical study, *BMC, Reproductive Biology and Endocrinology*, 2004. Available at: rbej.biomedcentral.com/articles/10.1186/1477-7827-2-58

4. Perry, A., Stephanou, A., Rayman, M. P., Dietary factors that affect the risk of pre-eclampsia, *BMJ Nutrition, Prevention & Health*, 2022, 5

5. Diguisto, C. et al, Maternal mortality in eight European countries with enhanced surveillance systems: Descriptive population based study, *BMJ*, 2022. Available at: www.bmj.com/content/379/bmj-2022-070621

6. Neu, J., Rushing, J., Caesarean versus vaginal delivery: Long-term infant outcomes and the hygiene hypothesis. *Clin. Perinatol.*, Jun. 2011, 38 (2), 321–31

7. Zhou, L., Qiu, W., Wang, J., Effects of vaginal microbiota transfer on the neurodevelopment and microbiome of caesarean-born infants: A blinded randomized controlled trial, *Cell Host & Microbe*, 2023, 31 (7), 1232–47.e5.

8. Future Market Insights (2023), Infant formula market is ready to rise at 8.5% CAGR due to adoption of baby milk escalates exponentially, Report by Future Market Insights Inc. Available at: www.globenewswire.com/en/news-release/2023/02/27/2615654/0/en/Infant-Formula-Market-is-Ready-to-Rise-at-8-5-CAGR-Due-to-Adoption-of-Baby-Milk-Escalates-Exponentially-Report-by-Future-Market-Insights-Inc.html [Accessed 14 Dec. 2023]

9. Neves, P. A. R., Vaz, J. S., Maia, F. S. et al, Rates and time trends in the consumption of breastmilk, formula and animal milk by children younger than 2 years from 2000 to 2019: Analysis of 113 countries, *The Lancet*, 2021. Available at: www.thelancet.com/journals/lanchi/article/PIIS2352-4642(21)00163-2/fulltext

10. World Health Organisation, Exclusive breastfeeding under 6 months: Data by country, 2022. Available at: apps.who.int/gho/data/view.main.NUT1730. [Accessed 14 Dec. 2023]

11. Iacobucci, G., Ultraprocessed food: Report calls for action to reduce levels in infant and baby food, *BMJ*, 2023, 381, 1318

12. Scarpone, R., Kimkool, P., Ierodiakonou, D. et al, Timing of allergenic food introduction and risk of immunoglobulin e–mediated food allergy: A systematic review and meta-analysis, *JAMA Pediatr.*, 2023, 177 (5), 489–97

13. Wallén, E., Auvinen, P., Kaminen-Ahola, N., The effects of early prenatal alcohol exposure on epigenome and embryonic development, *Genes*, 2021, 12 (7), 1095

14. James, J. E., Maternal caffeine consumption and pregnancy outcomes: a narrative review with implications for advice to mothers and mothers-to-be, *BMJ Evidence-Based Medicine*, 2021, 26, 114–15

Part 2. The Rollercoaster Years: Puberty and Adolescence

1. Greene, M. F., Samuel, L., 30 years ago, Romania deprived thousands of babies of human contact, *The Atlantic*, 2020. Available at: www.theatlantic.com/magazine/archive/2020/07/can-an-unloved-child-learn-to-love/612253/ [Accessed 14 Dec. 2023]

2. van de Pavert, S., Mebius, R., New insights into the development of lymphoid tissues, *Nat. Rev. Immunol.*, 2010, 10, 664–674

3. Klose, C. S. N., Artis, D., Innate lymphoid cells control signaling circuits to regulate tissue-specific immunity, *Cell Res.*, 2020, 30, 475–91. Available at: doi.org/10.1038/s41422-020-0323-8

4. World Bank, (n.d.) Prevalence of stunting, height for age (% of children under 5) – United Kingdom. Available at: data.worldbank.org/indicator/SH.STA.STNT.ZS?locations=GB&most_recent_value_desc=true [Accessed 14 Dec. 2023]

5. North/South Ireland food consumption survey: Summary report, 2001. Available at www.lenus.ie/handle/10147/265434

6. Marciano, L., Camerini, A., Morese, R., The developing brain in the digital era: a scoping review of structural and functional correlates of screen time in adolescence, *Frontiers in Psychology*, 2021, 12

7. Scamp: Study of cognition, adolescents and mobile phones, (n.d.). Available at: scampstudy.org/. [Accessed 14 Dec. 2023]

8. Anastasiadis, X., Matsas, A., Panoskaltsis, T. et al, Impact of chemicals on the age of menarche: A literature review, *Children*, 2023, 10 (7), 1234

9. Balaji, R., Subramanian, V. Meenakshi, Vijayakrishnan, G., Study on age of menarche between generations and the factors associated with it, *Clinical Epidemiology and Global Health*, 2021, 11, 100758

10. Schoenaker, D. , Mishra, G., Association between age at menarche and gestational diabetes mellitus: The Australian longitudinal study on women's health, *American Journal of Epidemiology*, 1 Apr. 2017, 185 (7), 554–61

11. Choudhury, Nishat, Research finds that 97% of women in the UK have been sexually harassed, in *Open Access Government*, 2022. Available at: www.openaccessgovernment.org/97-of-women-in-the-uk/105940/ [Accessed 14 Dec. 2023]

12. Stevens, G. A. et al, National, regional, and global estimates of anaemia by severity in women and children for 2000–19: a pooled analysis of population-representative data, *Lancet Global Health*, 2022, 10, e627–39.

13. World Health Organization, Anaemia in women and children, 2021. Available at: www.who.int/data/gho/data/themes/topics/anaemia_in_women_and_children

14. Munro, M. G., Heavy menstrual bleeding, iron deficiency, and iron deficiency anemia: Framing the issue, *Int. J. Gynecol. Obstet.*, 2023, 162 (2) 7–13.

15. Kessler, R. C., Berglund, P., Demler, O. et al, Lifetime prevalence and age-of-onset distributions of DSM-IV disorders in the national comorbidity survey replication. *Arch. Gen. Psychiatry*, 2005, 62 (6), 593–602.

Part 3. The Circles of Life: Adulting

1. Royal College of Psychiatrists, Hospital admissions for eating disorders increased by 84% in the last five years, 2022. Available at: www.rcpsych.ac.uk/news-and-features/latest-news/detail/2022/05/18/hospital-admissions-for-eating-disorders-increased-by-84-in-the-last-five-years [Accessed 15 Dec. 2023]

2. Riaz, M. N., Asif, M., Ali, R., Stability of vitamins during extrusion, *Crit. Rev. Food Sci. Nutr.*, Apr. 2009, 49 (4), 361–8

3. Via, M., The malnutrition of obesity: micronutrient deficiencies that promote diabetes. *ISRN Endocrinol.*, 2012, 2012, 103472

4. Spector, D, The odds of you being alive are incredibly small, 2012. Available at: www.businessinsider.com/infographic-the-odds-of-being-alive-2012-6?r=US&IR=T [Accessed 14 Dec. 2023]

5. Harris, I. D., Fronczak, C., Roth, L. et al, Fertility and the aging male. *Rev. Urol.*, 2011, 13 (4) e184–90

6. Watkins, A. J., Rubini, E., Hosier, E. D. et al, Paternal programming of offspring health, *Early Human Development*, 2020, 150, 105185

7. Gov.uk., Maternity pay and leave, (n.d.). Available at: www.gov.uk/maternity-pay-leave/pay#:~:text=Statutory%20Maternity%20Pay%20(%20SMP%20)%20is,for%20the%20next%2033%20weeks [Accessed 15 Dec. 2023]

8. United Nations Population Fund, Nearly half of all pregnancies are unintended – a global crisis, says new UNFPA report, 2022. Available at: www.unfpa.org/press/nearly-half-all-pregnancies-are-unintended-global-crisis-says-new-unfpa-report [Accessed 15 Dec. 2023]

9. Gov.uk., Health matters: reproductive health and pregnancy planning, (n.d.). Available at: www.gov.uk/government/publications/health-matters-reproductive-health-and-pregnancy-planning/health-matters-reproductive-health-and-pregnancy-planning [Accessed 15 Dec. 2023]

10. Office for National Statistics, Sexual offences victim characteristics, England and Wales: Year ending March 2022, 2023. Available at: www.ons.gov.uk/peoplepopulationandcommunity/crimeandjustice/articles/sexualoffencesvictimcharacteristicsenglandandwales/yearendingmarch2022#:~:text=In%20the%20year%20ending%20March%202022%2C%203.9%25%20of%20women%20and,March%202020%20(Figure%202) [Accessed 15 Dec. 2023]

11. Atella, V., Piano Mortari, A., Kopinska, J. et al, Trends in age-related disease burden and healthcare utilization. *Aging Cell.*, Feb. 2019 18 (1), e12861

12. Appiah, D., Nwabuo, C. C., Ebong, I. A. et al, Trends in age at natural menopause and reproductive life span among US women, 1959–2018. *JAMA*, 2021, 325 (13), 1328–30

13. Choe, S. A., Sung, J., Trends of premature and early menopause: A comparative study of the US national health and nutrition examination survey and the Korea national health and nutrition examination survey, *J. Korean Med. Sci.*, 13 Apr. 2020, 35 (14), e97

Part 4. *Avoiding the Twilight Zone: Building Your Health Span*

1. Ford, E. S., Bergmann, M. M., Kröger, J. et al, Healthy living is the best revenge: Findings from the European prospective investigation into cancer and nutrition-Potsdam study, *Arch. Intern. Med.*, 10 Aug 2009, 169 (15),1355–62
2. *The Lancet,* Menopause [series], in *Diabetes & Endocrinology,* 2022. Available at: www.thelancet.com/series/menopause [Accessed 15 Dec. 2023]
3. Bermingham, K. et al, Menopause is associated with post-prandial metabolism, metabolic health and lifestyle: The ZOE PREDICT study. *eBioMedicine,* 2022, 85, 104303.
4. Menstrual Migraine Centre, Menstrual migraine: A national migraine centre factsheet, (n.d.). Available at: www.national-migrainecentre.org.uk/understanding-migraine/factsheets-and-resources/menstrual-migraine/ [Accessed 14 Dec. 2023]
5. Blell, M., Grandmother hypothesis, grandmother effect, and residence patterns. In Callan, H., (Ed.), *The International Encyclopedia of Anthropology,* 2017, 1–5
6. Tiplady, B., Amati, F., Dunn, C. et al, Alcohol and memory: A selective reminding word-number test administered on a mobile phone, *Journal of Psychopharmacology,* 2009, 63, A72
7. Gould, D. C., Petty, R., Jacobs, H. S., The male menopause – does it exist? For and against, *BMJ,* 2000. Available at: www.ncbi.nlm.nih.gov/pmc/articles/PMC1127205/#:~:text=

The%20term%20"male%20menopause"%20is,production
%20and%20plasma%20concentrations%20fall.

8. NHS, The male menopause, 2022. Available at: www.nhs.uk/
conditions/male-menopause/#:~:text=If%20the%20
specialist%20confirms%20this,an%20injection%20or%20
a%20gel. [Accessed 14 Dec. 2023]

9. Vallat, R., Berry, S. E., Tsereteli, N. et al, How people wake up
is associated with previous night's sleep together with physical
activity and food intake, *Nature Communications*, 2022, 13, 7116

10. Furman, D., Campisi, J., Verdin, E. et al, Chronic inflammation in the etiology of disease across the life span. *Nat. Med.,
2019*, 25, 1822–32

11. Cooper, J., Pastorello, Y., Slevin, M. A., Meta-analysis investigating the relationship between inflammation in autoimmune
disease, elevated CRP, and the risk of dementia, *Front Immunol.,* 27 Jan. 2023, 14, 1087571

12. Mazidi, M., Valdes, A. M., Ordovas, J. M. et al, Meal-induced
inflammation: postprandial insights from the Personalised
Responses to Dietary Composition Trial (PREDICT) study in
1000 participants. *Am. J. Clin. Nutr.* 2021 Sep 1;114(3):1028–38.

13. Bermingham, K. M., May, A., Asnicar, F. et al, Snack quality
and snack timing are associated with cardiometabolic blood
markers: the ZOE PREDICT study, *European Journal of
Nutrition*, 2023. Available at: link.springer.com/art-
icle/10.1007/s00394-023-03241-6

14. NHS Better Health, Self-help CBT techniques. Available at:
www.nhs.uk/every-mind-matters/mental-wellbeing-tips/
self-help-cbt-techniques/

15. Williams, M., Penman, D. *Mindfulness: A practical guide to finding
peace in a frantic world*, Piatkus Books, 2011

16. Derakhshandeh-Rishehri, S-M., Kazemi, A., Shim, S. R. et al,
Effect of olive oil phenols on oxidative stress biomarkers:

A systematic review and dose-response meta-analysis of randomized clinical trials. *Food Science & Nutrition*, 2023. Available at: www.ncbi.nlm.nih.gov/pmc/articles/PMC10171518/

17. Valdes, A. M., Walter, J., Segal, E. et al, Role of the gut microbiota in nutrition and health, *BMJ*, 2018, 361, k2179

18. Parker, A., Romano, S., Ansorge, R. et al, Fecal microbiota transfer between young and aged mice reverses hallmarks of the aging gut, eye, and brain, *Microbiome*, 2022, 10, 68

19. Dongyue, L., Lanrong, C., Yanhong, G. et al, Fecal microbiota transplantation improves intestinal inflammation in mice with ulcerative colitis by modulating intestinal flora composition and down-regulating NF-kB signaling pathway, *Microbial Pathogenesis*, 2022, 173 (A), 105803, ISSN 0882-4010

20. Bosco, N., Noti, M., The aging gut microbiome and its impact on host immunity, *Genes & Immunity*, 2021, 22, 289–303

21. Dattani, S., Spooner, F., Ritchie, H. et al Causes of Death, OurWorldInData.org, 2023. Retrieved from: ourworldindata. org/causes-of-death

22. Manson, B., Welcome to the VITAL Study. Available at: www.vitalstudy.org/index.html [Accessed 14 Dec. 2023]

23. O'Connor, E. A., Evans, C. V., Ivlev, I. et al, Vitamin and mineral supplements for the primary prevention of cardiovascular disease and cancer: Updated evidence report and systematic review for the US Preventive Services Task Force', *JAMA*, 2022, 327(23), 2334–47

24. Murray, C. J. L. et al, Global burden of 87 risk factors in 204 countries and territories, 1990–2019: A systematic analysis for the Global Burden of Disease Study 2019, *The Lancet*, 2020, 396, 1223–49

25. UN WPP (2022); HMD (2023); Zijdeman et al (2015); Riley (2005). Available at: ourworldindata.org/grapher/life-expectancy?tab=map [Accessed 14 Dec. 2023]

26. Statista, Age-specific death rate per 1,000 population in the United Kingdom in 2021, by gender, 2022. Available at: www.statista.com/statistics/1125118/death-rate-united-kingdom-uk-by-age/ [Accessed 14 Dec. 2023]

27. World Health Organization, Global report on hypertension: the race against a silent killer, 2023. Available at: www.who.int/southeastasia/publications/i/item/9789240081062 [Accessed 14 Dec. 2023]

28. Cancer Research, Cancer incidence statistics, (n.d). Available at: www.cancerresearchuk.org/health-professional/cancer-statistics/incidence [Accessed 15 Dec. 2023]

29. Cancer Research, Cancer survival statistics, (n.d). Available at: www.cancerresearchuk.org/health-professional/cancer-statistics/survival#:~:text=More%20than%2080%25%20of%20people,more%20(2010%2D11) [Accessed 15 Dec. 2023]

30. Cancer Research, Statistics by cancer type, (n.d). Available at: www.cancerresearchuk.org/health-professional/cancer-statistics/statistics-by-cancer-type [Accessed 15 Dec. 2023]

31. World Health Organization, Preventing cancer, (n.d). Available at: www.who.int/activities/preventing-cancer#:~:text=Between%2030%E2%80%9350%25%20of%20all,for%20the%20control%20of%20cancer [Accessed 15 Dec. 2023]

32. Stride Foundation, Helping people walk away from addiction [landing page], (n.d). Available at: stridefoundation.com [Accessed 15 Dec. 2023]

33. Nutt, D., Equasy – An overlooked addiction with implications for the current debate on drug harms, *Journal of Psychopharmacology*, 2009, 23 (1), 3–5

34. Hope, C., Ecstasy: No more dangerous than horse riding, *Telegraph*. Available at: www.telegraph.co.uk/news/uknews/law-and-order/4537874/Ecstasy-no-more-dangerous-than-horse-riding.html [Accessed 15 Dec. 2023]

35. Nutt, D. J., King, L. A., Phillips, L. D., Drug harms in the UK: A multicriteria decision analysi, *The Lancet*, 2010, 376, 1558–65

36. Papadimitriou, N., Markozannes, G., Kanellopoulou, A. et al, An umbrella review of the evidence associating diet and cancer risk at 11 anatomical sites, *Nature Communications*, 2021, 12, 4579

37. World Cancer Research Fund/American Institute for Cancer Research, Continuous project Update Project Expert Report 2018. Meat, fish and dairy products and the risk of cancer, 2018. Available at: www.wcrf.org/wp-content/uploads/2021/02/Meat-fish-and-dairy-products.pdf [Accessed 15 Dec. 2023]

38. World Health Organization, Human cancer: Known causes and prevention by organ site IARC monographs on the identification of carcinogenic hazards to humans and handbooks of cancer prevention [monographs], 2019. Downloaded from: https://monographs.iarc.who.int/wp-content/uploads/2019/12/OrganSitePoster.PlusHandbooks.pdf. [Accessed 15th December 2023.]

39. Bolte, L.A., Lee, K. A., Björk, J. R. et al, Association of a Mediterranean diet with outcomes for patients treated with immune checkpoint blockade for advanced melanoma, *JAMA Oncol.*, 1 May 2023, 9 (5), 705–9

40. Amati, F., McCann, L., Castañeda-Gutiérrez, E. et al, Infant fat mass and later child and adolescent health outcomes: A systematic review. *Arch. Dis. Child.*, 8 Nov. 2023, archdischild-2023-325798

41. Wood, R., Anthropometric measurements of 100m olympic champions, Topend Sports Website, Dec. 2015, www.topend-sports.com/events/summer/science/athletics-100m.htm [Accessed 15 Dec. 2023]

42. National Institute for Health and Care Excellence, Keep the size of your waist to less than half of your height, updated NICE draft guideline recommends, 2022. Available at: www.

nice.org.uk/news/article/keep-the-size-of-your-waist-to-less-than-half-of-your-height-updated-nice-draft-guideline-recommends [Accessed 15 Dec. 2023]

43. Ross, R., Neeland, I. J., Yamashita, S. et al, Waist circumference as a vital sign in clinical practice: A Consensus Statement from the IAS and ICCR Working Group on Visceral Obesity. *Nat. Rev. Endocrinol.*, 2020, 16, 177–89

Part 5. To Longevity, and Beyond!

1. AARP, Second Half of Life Study, 2022. Available at: www.aarp.org/content/dam/aarp/research/surveys_statistics/life-leisure/2022/second-half-life-desires-concerns-report.doi.10.26419-2Fres.00538.001.pdf [Accessed 15 Dec. 2023]

2. Galambos, N. L., Krahn, H. J., Johnson, M. D., The U shape of happiness across the life course: Expanding the discussion, *Perspect Psychol. Sci.*, Jul 2020, 15 (4), 898–912. doi: 10.1177/1745691620902428.

3. Fadnes, L. T., Økland, J. M., Haaland, Ø. A. et al, Correction: Estimating impact of food choices on life expectancy: A modeling study, *PLOS Medicine*, 2022, 19 (3), e1003962.

4. PriorityApp, Food for healthy life, (n.d.). Available at: priorityapp.shinyapps.io/Food/ [Accessed 15 Dec. 2023]

5. World Health Organization, Preventing cancer, (n.d.). Available at: www.who.int/activities/preventing-cancer#:~:text=Between%2030%E2%80%9350%25%20of%20all,for%20the%20control%20of%20cancer [Accessed 15 Dec. 2023]

6. Cudejko, T., Gardiner, J., Akpan, A. et al, Minimal shoes improve stability and mobility in persons with a history of falls, *Sci. Rep.*, 2020, 10, 21755

7. Bauer, A. Z., Swan, S. H., Kriebel, D. et al, Paracetamol use during pregnancy – a call for precautionary action, *Nat. Rev. Endocrinol.*, 2021, 17, 757–766

8. King's College London, Our people: Professor Claire Steeves, (n.d.). Available at: www.kcl.ac.uk/people/claire-steves [Accessed 15 Dec. 2023]

9. Ni Lochlainn, M., Bowyer, R. C. E., Steves, C. J., Dietary protein and muscle in aging people: The potential role of the gut microbiome, *Nutrients*, 20 Jul. 2018, 10 (7) 929

10. World Health Organization, The Top 10 causes of death, 2020. Available at: www.who.int/news-room/fact-sheets/detail/the-top-10-causes-of-death

11. World Health Organization Dementia, (n.d.). Available at: www.who.int/news-room/fact-sheets/detail/dementia/?gclid=CjwKCAjwkNOpBhBEEiwAb3MvvYX_JDY-DoLPsEhAlTM4ozC-t_o3brK73y2XyCK66zGioY6WQ32rOBoCvggQAvD_BwE [Accessed 15 Dec. 2023]

12. World Health Organization Dementia, (n.d.). Available at: www.who.int/news-room/fact-sheets/detail/dementia/?gclid=CjwKCAjwkNOpBhBEEiwAb3MvvYX_JDY-DoLPsEhAlTM4ozC-t_o3brK73y2XyCK66zGioY6WQ32rOBoCvggQAvD_BwE [Accessed 15 Dec. 2023]

Part 6. Health is the New Wealth: This is How You Get Rich

1. Doll, R., Bradford Hill, A., Lung cancer and other causes of death in relation to smoking, *Br. Med. J.*, 10 Nov. 1956, 2 (5001), 1071–81.

2. Directorate-General for Agriculture and Rural Development 92–22, Monitoring EU agri-food trade: Developments in

2022. Available at: agriculture.ec.europa.eu/system/files/
2023-04/monitoring-agri-food-trade_dec2022_en.pdf
[Accessed 15 Dec. 2023]

3. Dray, S., In focus: Food waste in the UK, 2021. Available at:
lordslibrary.parliament.uk/food-waste-in-the-uk/ [Accessed
15 Dec. 2023]

4. Jacka, F. N., O'Neil, A., Opie, R. et al, A randomised controlled trial of dietary improvement for adults with major
depression (the 'SMILES' trial), *BMC Medicine,* 2017, 15 (23)

5. Cryan, J. F., O'Riordan, K. J., Cowan, C. S. M. et al, The
microbiota-gut-brain axis, *Physiological Reviews,* 2019, 99 (4)
1877–2013

6. Berry, S.E., Valdes, A. M., Drew, D. A. et al, Human postprandial responses to food and potential for precision nutrition.
Nat. Med., 2020, 26, 964–73

7. Yeoh, Y. K., Zuo, T, Lui, G. C. et al, Gut microbiota composition reflects disease severity and dysfunctional immune
responses in patients with COVID-19, *Gut,* 2021, 70, 698–706

8. Bermingham, K. M., Linenberg, I., Polidori, L. et al,
Improved cardiometabolic health using a personalized
nutrition approach: the ZOE METHOD study, *MDPI,*
2023. Available at: www.mdpi.com/2504-3900/91/1/55

9. O'Donnell, M. P., Fox, B. W., Chao, P. H. et al, A neurotransmitter produced by gut bacteria modulates host sensory
behaviour, *Nature,* 2020, 583, 415–20

10. Dinan, T. G., Stilling, R. M., Stanton, C. et al, Collective
unconscious: How gut microbes shape human behavior,
Journal of Psychiatric Research, 2015, 63,1–9, ISSN 0022-3956.

11. McGuinness, A., Davis, J. A., Dawson, S. L. et al, A systematic review of gut microbiota composition in observational
studies of major depressive disorder, bipolar disorder and
schizophrenia, *Mol. Psychiatry,* 2022, 27, 1920–35

12. Butler, M. I., Bastiaanssen, T. F. S., Long-Smith, C. et al, The gut microbiome in social anxiety disorder: evidence of altered composition and function. *Transl. Psychiatry*, 2023, 13, 95
13. Valdes, A. M., Walter, J., Segal, E. et al, Role of the gut microbiota in nutrition and health, *BMJ*, 2018, 361, k2179
14. Deakin University, Alfred Deakin Professor Felice Jacka, (n.d.). Available at: www.deakin.edu.au/research/researcher-stories/professor-felice-jacka. [Accessed 15 Dec. 2023]

Glossary

Bacteria: small microbes that are present almost everywhere, including our bodies.

Blue Zones: the regions of the world where people live the longest, including Japan, Greece and Italy, where habits tend to consist of a plant-based diet, low alcohol intake and daily exercise.

BMI (Body mass index): a well-known formula to estimate body fat by dividing your weight (in kilogrammes) by height (in metres) squared. Whilst a simple proxy, it is unable to differentiate between fat and muscle.

Carcinogen: a substance with the ability to cause cancer in living cells.

Co-enzyme: organic compounds required by enzymes to function.

Conception: the act of being conceived/fertilization.

Eclampsia: a rare but life-threatening medical condition occurring usually in the second half of pregnancy, where a woman experiences seizures or coma.

EDCs (Endocrine-Disrupting Chemicals): these can be natural or industrial chemicals which interfere with the body's hormones and can cause subsequent health problems.

Endometrium/endometrial lining: one of the layers of uterus tissue which is controlled by female sex hormones. This is the lining that is shed, causing bleeding, during a menstrual period.

Enzymes: proteins that start, or speed up, reactions.

Epidemiology: the study of populations in order to discover the causes of disease.

First 1,000 days: a window of opportunity between conception and a child's second birthday where their brain, body and immune system experience significant development.

GDM (Gestational diabetes mellitus): a medical condition affecting about 5 per cent of pregnancies where blood sugar is high (glucose). Whilst this usually disappears after birth, it poses risks to both mother (for example, future diabetes risk) and baby (for example, being large for gestational age, congenital malformations, breathing problems).

Genes: a small group of chemicals on our DNA which coordinate how our bodies make proteins. There are around 20,000 in each cell.

Glucocorticoids: a naturally occurring steroid hormone which has an essential role in controlling sugar levels (glucose), protein and fat metabolism in our bodies.

Gonadal steroid hormones: sex hormones produced in the gonads (ovaries in females and testes in males).

HGH (Human growth hormone): a hormone essential for growth, particularly in childhood, produced from a pea-sized gland (pituitary) in the base of our brains.

Hormones: chemicals which coordinate and signal functions in our bodies – they tell our bodies the whats and whens of life.

Hyperemesis Gravidarum (HG): when morning sickness is so intractable it leads to weight loss, dehydration and electrolyte imbalance. It can need treatment in hospital with anti-sickness medication and fluids.

Hypoallergenic: something which is unlikely to cause allergy, often used to describe certain dog breeds or plant types.

Insulin: the hormone which responds to high blood sugar (glucose) and brings levels down by converting it to glycogen (energy stores) in the liver and fat cells.

Lactobacillus: a bacterium that is present in many foods such as yoghurt, cheese and pickles. It breaks down lactose in milk and other sugars into lactic acid, which helps to preserve the food and adjusts its acidity.

Maternal microbiome: the microbiome blueprint found in a pregnant woman's gut and vagina which becomes the initial blueprint for the baby's gut microbiome. Its composition is also thought to impact pregnancy outcomes and risk of pre-term labour.

Metabolism: the way our bodies use and make energy, which can vary with a variety of factors such as physical activity, temperature and illness.

Microbiome: all the biological species making up a community. We have numerous different microbiomes in the human body.

Parasite: an organism that survives by using another species (the host).

Pituitary gland: a pea-sized gland at the base of our brains which produces essential hormones for our bodies to function.

Pre-eclampsia: a medical condition in pregnancy where blood pressure is high (hypertension) and there is protein in the urine (proteinuria). If untreated it can lead to eclampsia, which is life-threatening.

Prolactin: a hormone which triggers milk production/lactation and develops breast tissue in mammals.

UPF – Ultra-Processed Foods: foods made with industrial processes that have added ingredients and chemicals which would not be found in a home kitchen, including emulsifiers, artificial sweeteners, colouring, flavourings and modified starches. They are hyperpalatable, low in beneficial nutrients and fibre, and high in energy. They are associated with negative overall health when eaten regularly.

Viruses: the smallest microbes which are mostly harmless but can cause problems too. They can live in our bodies and have a healthy role.

ZOE: a data-science personalized nutrition and health company which I work for, whose mission is to improve the health of millions.

Further Resources
for Curious Bodies

Five Books
- *Food for Life: Your Guide to the New Science of Eating Well*, Professor Tim Spector
- *Ultra-Processed People: Why do we all eat stuff that isn't food . . . and why can't we stop?*, Dr Chris van Tulleken
- *The Body Keeps the Score*, Dr Bessel van der Kolk
- *Bad Science*, Dr Ben Goldacre
- *The Well-Lived Life*, Dr Gladys McGarey

Five Favourite ZOE Podcasts:
- 'How to maximize health in your later years'
- 'Gut microbiome testing: What can it reveal about your health?'
- 'Why unhealthy carbs are making you sick, and what to do about it'
- 'How body fat impacts health and ageing'
- 'The shocking way ultra-processed foods damage your brain'

Five Instagram handles to follow:
- Dr Sarah Berry – @drsarahberry
- Dr Tim Spector – @tim.spector
- Zoe – @zoe
- Dr Will Bulsiewicz – @theguthealthmd
- Dr Karan Rajan – @drkaranrajan

Five Documentaries:
- *BBC Maestro*: Tim Spector, 'The Science of Eating Well'
- *You Are What You Eat: A Twin Experiment* (Netflix), 2024
- *Fed Up* (directed by Stephanie Soechtig), 2014
- *Food, Inc.* (directed by Robert Kenner), 2008
- Davina McCall: *Sex, Myths and the Menopause*, Channel 4, 2021

Acknowledgements

Thank you so much to the people that made this book possible. First of all my family, who are not only my bedrock and inspiration but also the fuel that helps my creative fire to burn. My husband Paul Sculfor and my wonderful mamma for supporting me with writing on weekends and late into the night.

My brilliant editor at Penguin Michael Joseph, Karolina Kaim, who gave me carte blanche to write the book I wanted to write, and the rest of the MJ team who sprang into action to make it a reality. My Greek goddess big sister Georgie Wolfinden whose brilliant PR skills secured me the press article that inspired Karolina to contact me. My right-hand woman Dr Lucy McCann, without whom I would not have finished the book in time, and the irreplaceable Emma who keeps me sane alongside Cristina, our magical nanny.

Thank you to Tim Newman for jumping on and helping me demystify some of the more complex science to make it more accessible. Thank you to my wonderful agent Amanda Harris for championing me and being there for my ideas at 9 p.m. on a Sunday. Thank you to my brilliant ZOE team for supporting my work and growing with me; especially to Tim

Spector for helping me grow as an author and as a science communicator.

Last but definitely not least, huge thanks to my clients, my friends, my students and those who I've spoken to at talks and events. Your unique human stories and interest in these topics are what shapes my passion for communicating science.

Illustration Credits

1. Chart courtesy of Tyler Vigen
2. iStock.com/DmytroDonets
3. iStock.com/Bezvershenko
4. © Fondazione Barilla
5. Illustration 71548656 © Alla72 | Dreamstime.com
7. © 2020 Jansen, C. H. J. R., Kastelein, A. W., Kleinrouweler, E., Van Leeuwen, E., De Jong, K. H., Pajkrt, E., Van Noorden, C. J. F., *Acta Obstetricia et Gynecologica Scandinavica,* published by John Wiley & Sons Ltd on behalf of Nordic Federation of Societies of Obstetrics and Gynecology (NFOG)
11. © 2016 Dulac, C., Autry, A. E, Kohl, J., *BioEssays*, published by WILEY Periodicals, Inc.
13. WHO *(2019),* ourworldindata.org/grapher/number-of-deaths-by-risk-factor?country=~European+Region+%28WHO%29, published online at OurWorldInData.org. Retrieved from: ourworldindata.org/global-rise-of-education
16. © 2015 © SAGE Publications
19. Figure adapted from © 2023, Lars T. Fadnes, L. T., Celis-Morales, C., Økland, J., Parra-Soto, S, Livingstone, K. M., Ho, F. K., Pell, J. P., Balakrishna, R., Arjmand, E. J., Johansson, K. E., Haaland, Ø. A., Mathers, J. C.

22. © 2020 WHO, The top 10 causes of death, WHO Global Health Estimates

Every effort has been made to ensure images are correctly attributed, however if any omission or error has been made, please notify the publisher for correction in future editions.

Index